A Complete Guide To

Understanding, Managing

&

Improving Your Peripheral Neuropathy

By Michael Veselak, DC, BCIM, CFMP

Preface and Disclaimer

The information contained in this book is a small piece of 35 years of clinical practice, learning from other doctors that paved my way and patients who share their stories. This is, in no way, a complete work on the subject but rather a handbook or guide for those who suffer from this disease to search for the answers. I am simply conveying information and opinion; this is not a substitute for medical care. All information in this book is NOT a substitute for standard medical care. Please consult your physician before considering any information in this book. This book is an opinion, not a protocol. It is the reader's responsibility to seek appropriate medical care, and to understand that this book does not suggest or imply that treating neuropathy is anything but reserved for appropriate medical establishments.

Table of Contents

PART ONE

THE EVALUATION

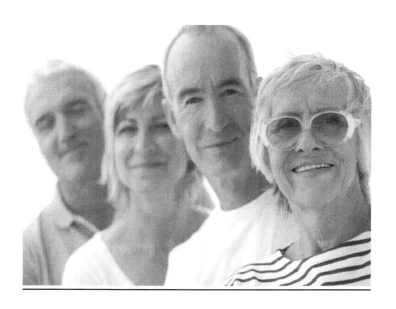

Chapter One
I Am Not Alone

Finally, after 16 months of evaluations and various doctors, Richard received his diagnosis. He was excited. Thoughts raced through his head. He looked forward to no more restless nights, no more cramping, and no more tingling and numbness. He could, once again, enjoy the little things such as taking his dogs for a walk. **"Peripheral Neuropathy"**, the neurologist confidently stated.

Peripheral Neuropathy had controlled his thoughts, his actions and, virtually, his life for the past 16 months. When his wife discussed traveling now that he retired, he was scared that he could not walk the distances traveling would require. Richard found himself making excuses to his friends about why he could not play in his weekly golf game. There was no way he could walk the course with them as he would suffer too much that night.

"What does this mean?", he asked the neurologist.

The doctor began to explain as the name suggests, it is a nerve condition that affects the nerves away from the center or away from the spinal cord. "Neuro" means nerve and "pathy" means condition. It is quite common. In fact, it affects globally hundreds of millions of people. It has been estimated that 3 - 4% of people over the age of 55 have some form of peripheral neuropathy. There are over 20 million people affected in America.

As the doctor continued, Richard was half listening as his thoughts carried him to another place. How is it that so many people are affected, and I hardly know anything about it? Why did so many other doctors not understand or know how to help me?

"Could you write that diagnosis down for me, doctor, as my memory is not quite as good as it used to be? I would like to read more about it and tell my wife

Michael came to our clinic with pain and numbness in his feet, which he had experienced for the past 3 years. He was only 42, overweight and depressed. The pain in his feet were so severe and he was unable to work anymore. In fact, he had to wear a spinal stimulator to help control that level of pain. After our evaluation, I reviewed his medical records including nerve studies and lab panels from his neurologist. I explained to Michael about the complexities of treating peripheral neuropathy primarily because no two people are alike in the causation. We implemented our peripheral neuropathy treatment recovery program, and with the help of our physical therapist, within a few visits, his level of pain diminished considerably. He told us that he turned his spinal stimulator off as he no longer needed it to control the pain. Michael can now exercise, walk and basically resume a normal life. He has lost approximately 55 pounds, and recently following a consultation with his doctors, he stopped taking the entire list of medications. He is grateful for the care he has received and thanked us for changing his life.

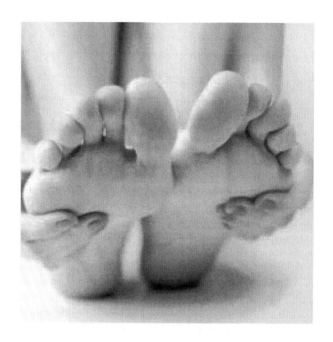

Chapter Two
The First Step

When Richard arrived home, he shared with his wife his diagnosis and showed her the prescription for the medication that should resolve his symptoms.

Together, they sat at the computer and began to read about Peripheral Neuropathy.

The nervous system is divided into two main parts. The central part, which is the brain along with the spinal cord and the peripheral nervous system. The peripheral nervous system extends from the brain and spinal cord, and connects the rest of our body. It connects our skin, eyes, mouth, internal organs, hands, feet, arms and legs.

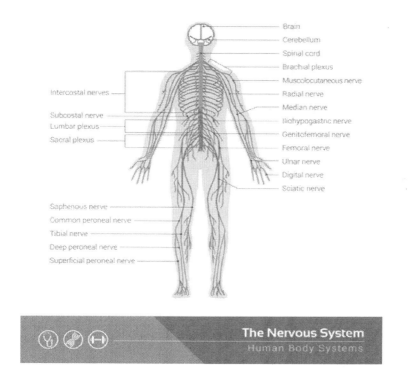

Intercostal nerves

Subcostal nerve
Lumbar plexus
Sacral plexus

Saphenous nerve
Common peroneal nerve
Tibial nerve
Deep peroneal nerve
Superficial peroneal nerve

Brain
Cerebellum
Spinal cord
Brachial plexus
Muscolocutaneous nerve
Radial nerve
Median nerve
Iliohypogastric nerve
Genitofemoral nerve
Femoral nerve
Ulnar nerve
Digital nerve
Sciatic nerve

The Nervous System
Human Body Systems

There are essentially *three types of peripheral nerves.* There are the *sensory nerves,* which extend from the various receptors in the body and send messages up the spinal cord to the brain. These receptors allow us to interpret or perceive if a body part is at rest or moving, if there is light touch, if it feels hot or cold, if there is vibration or tingling and numbness.

The *motor nerves* are the second type of peripheral nerves. These nerves send impulses down from the brain and spinal cord to all the muscles in the body. They control all our necessary movements such as walking, lifting, bending, moving and even movements with our hands such as grasping an object. If there is any damage to the motor nerves, it can exhibit weakness, cramping, or difficulty with movement.

The third type of peripheral nerves is the *autonomic nerve*. These nerves control involuntary activity such as heart rate, blood pressure and digestion. When these nerves are affected or damaged, one can experience hyperhidrosis or hypohidrosis (increase or decrease in sweating), increase or decrease in heart rate, digestive difficulties, diarrhea, constipation, abnormal pupil size or sexual dysfunction.

Basically, damage to the peripheral nervous system can impact all parts of your body from your eyes, ears, and skin to your muscles and including all your internal organs.

This, in part, is what makes it difficult to diagnose and why traditional treatments have not been entirely successful. Treatments, to date, have dealt with suppressing the symptoms, and not looking at the whole body and figuring out what caused the inflammation or the damage to the peripheral nerve in the first place.

Damage to any of these peripheral nerves interrupts communication between the brain and spinal cord, and the output of these nerves become affected. Sensations such as burning, numbness, tingling, pain or cramping can occur because of this damage, and the loss or lack of communication.

As he read more, Richard was well on the frustrating journey of discovering why his other doctors did not recognize this problem and why it is so difficult to treat.

How come they did not test him to determine if his electric wiring was breaking down and why his hands and feet were no longer communicating properly with his brain?

Like clockwork, he woke up at 2 am with the pain and burning sensation in his feet. This night, his legs seemed particularly more restless, with a cramping vise like sensation around his calves. As usual, he did not want to disturb his wife. So, he wandered the house searching for comfort and a little more rest.

As he sat in his favorite chair, Richard decided to continue to learn more about his condition.

TYPES OF PERIPHERAL NEUROPATHY

Currently, there are more than 100 types of peripheral neuropathy identified. They are classified according to the type of damage to the nerves.

To simplify, there are two general types of peripheral neuropathy. Mononeuropathy and Polyneuropathy.

Mononeuropathy, which affects one nerve at a time. Physical trauma such as an accident or repetitive trauma, are the most common causes. For example, carpal tunnel syndrome, which can occur from repetitive stress or repetitive motion affects the median nerve. This injury is prevalent amongst assembly line workers and individuals that use their keyboards for prolonged periods. The damage to the median nerve can result in numbness, tingling and pain on the first three fingers on the thumb side of the hand. It commonly becomes more pronounced at night while sleeping.

Another type of mononeuropathy is Bell's Palsy, which is a form of facial paralysis and can cause weakness or paralysis to one side of the face. This condition affects the seventh cranial nerve or facial nerve. The exact cause of this is unknown, but it is believed to be the result of inflammation, swelling or virus.

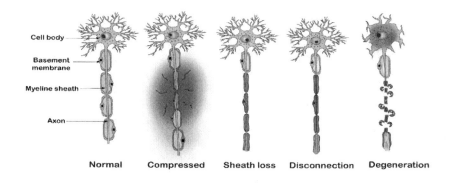

Other common examples of mononeuropathy that affect the hands and feet are:

Ulnar nerve palsy: This occurs when the nerve that passes close to the surface of the skin at the elbow gets damaged. Momentary irritation of this type of damage is more commonly known as "when   we hit our funny bone."

Radial Nerve Palsy: as known as Saturday night palsy which affects the radial nerve and causes weakness of the muscles of the wrist and forearm causing wrist drop.

Tarsal Tunnel: This injury, which is also known as posterior tibial neuralgia which is a compression type neuropathy. Patients that have this complain of numbness, pain or tingling on the first 3 toes of the foot.

Polyneuropathy is the most common form of peripheral neuropathy. It can be acute and / or chronic, generally slow developing over a long period of time. However, the symptoms can also occur suddenly.   It can affect the motor component, sensory and autonomic nerves individually, or a combination of all three.

The most common cause of polyneuropathy is from diabetes affecting millions of people.

As with all neuropathy symptoms, the evaluation must be thorough including a complete assessment of the neurological system, motor, sensory, and autonomic, and evaluating labs and physical examination findings.

The causes are vast. They could range from high blood sugar, heavy metal toxicity, Lyme's disease, abusive alcohol behavior, diabetes, autoimmune reactions, environmental toxins, cancer or chemo induced neuropathy. Poor nutrition, in particular B vitamin deficiency, can also lead to polyneuropathy.

Guillain Barre syndrome is one of the most serious polyneuropathies that can occur. It occurs when the body's immune system begins to attack the nerves in the body. The symptoms occur fast and, at times, can lead to paralysis. Early signs and symptoms include weakness and tingling. However, despite severity of the disease, recovery rates are good with early and appropriate support and treatment.

As he continued to read, Richard felt overwhelmed at how complex the nervous system is and how he took his health for granted.

Did he ignore the warning signs? What other parts of his body were affected?

Barbara, a 38 year old female, came to our office complaining of weakness, burning and pain in her hands and feet. She explained that the symptoms had been present for approximately 6 years and were progressing. Upon evaluation, it was noted that she had high arches and hammertoes. We sent her for some electro-diagnostic studies to include NCV and EMG along with a nerve biopsy. The neurologist confirmed the diagnosis of Charcot Marie Tooth. The emphasis on treatment was dietary and lifestyle changes to help control the symptoms and delay the progression. This included an autoimmune Paleo type diet, nutritional support and exercise in the form of swimming and resistance training. We also recommended that she continue with her Yoga and Meditation. In office, therapies were provided, initially, to work on balance, nerve activation and strength training. Barbara did very well with our treatment and was able to control her pain and minimize her flare-ups. Essentially, she resumed her normal daily activities.

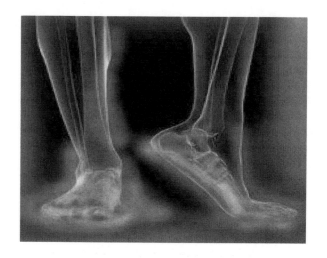

Chapter Three
Motor, Sensory and Autonomic
OH MY!

THE TEN MOST COMMON SIGNS OF PERIPHERAL NEUROPATHY

- *NUMBNESS*
- *BURNING FEET*
- *CRAMPING*
- *SHARP ELECTRIC PAIN*
- *PAIN WHEN WALKING*
- *DIFFICULTY SLEEPING FROM LEG DISCOMFORT*
- *PRICKLING/TINGLING FEELINGS*
- *LOSS OF BALANCE/ FALLING*
- *WEAKNESS*
- *SWELLING*

As we explained earlier, there are three types of nerves, sensory, motor and autonomic.

The symptoms we experience depend upon which nerves are affected. If the **sensory nerves** are affected, we will experience numbness, tingling, or electrical pains. Within the sensory nerves, there are small myelinated and unmyelinated sensory fibers that deal with pain and temperature. There are, also, large myelinated sensory fibers that deal with vibration and joint position sense.

Myelin is the insulation or the covering of the portion of the nerve which is called the axon. Its job is to increase the function of the nerve impulses. The myelin is comprised mostly of fat. This protective covering can become damaged by inflammation, which is common in Diabetes.

The brain and nerves require good fat. It provides protection, insulation and enhances overall function. It must be good fats which will be discussed later in the book.

The **motor nerves** help control muscle. If they are affected, they can cause cramping, weakness and loss of balance. These are large myelinated fibers.

The autonomic nerves carry information to our blood vessels. These are small myelinated and unmyelinated fibers. When they are affected, it can affect our blood pressure, heart rate, sweat and GI (gastrointestinal issues) like constipation or diarrhea.

Autonomic neuropathy is a group of symptoms that occur when there is damage to the nerves that manage every day body functions. Messages become affected from the brain stem which is the part of the brain that controls autonomic function and other organs, sweat glands or blood vessels.

The brain stem is supposed to be kept in check or inhibited by other parts or lobes of the brain. For many reasons when this becomes unchecked, symptoms of autonomic dysfunction or autonomic neuropathy can begin to occur.

Often, presentation of neuropathy includes a combination of motor, sensory and autonomic.

SYMPTOMS OF AUTONOMIC NEUROPATHY

Cardiovascular Symptoms:

1. Exercise Intolerance
2. Fatigue
3. Dizziness
4. Lightheadedness
5. Balance Issues

Gastrointestinal Symptoms:

1. Difficulty Swallowing
2. Bloating
3. Nausea
4. Vomiting
5. Constipation
6. Loss of Bowel Control

Genitourinary Symptoms:

1. Loss of Bladder Control
2. Urinary Tract Infections

3. Urinary Frequency
4. Erectile Dysfunction
5. Loss of Libido
6. Vaginal Dryness

Sweat Glands:

1. Itchy Skin
2. Dry Skin
3. Limb Hair Loss
4. Calluses

General Symptoms:

1. Difficulty Driving at Night
2. Depression
3. Anxiety
4. Sleep Disorders
5. Cognitive Changes

During the night when Richard began to experience that burning sensation in his feet that recently was keeping him awake at night, he understood now that his diabetes affected his motor, sensory and autonomic nerves.

Over the past few years, he would experience intermittent periods of tingling, numbness and occasional burning. As well, he was starting to get these cramps in his calf, primarily, at night. He also recalled buying insoles because the bottoms of his feet were sore from walking.

What he did not realize was that his occasional vertigo and balance issues along with the calluses on his feet and the loss of hair on his leg were also related to the neuropathy.

He was curious as to what tests the doctor was going to run and what other medications would be prescribed that would fix him. It had only been a few nights but the first medication has not helped. In fact, it has made him a little dizzy, clumsy and depressed.

Karen, a 32 year old female, was initially evaluated in our office with complaints of dizziness, nausea, bloating, anxiety, loss of balance, fatigue and a history of passing out. She had extreme pain in her legs and feet where the sensation of her clothes touching her skin would create pain. When we evaluated her labs, they were relatively normal. The neurologist she saw did the table tilt test for dysautonomia, which was also normal. We sent her for some labs to evaluate further what the underlying cause could be. Lab tests included Lyme's, chemical sensitivity, neurological autoimmunity, heavy metals, organic acids and hormone testing. We also ordered gluten sensitivity testing from Cyrex Labs. We left no stone unturned on trying to identify the root cause of this neuropathy. When we received the tests, they all came back normal except the gluten sensitivity test, which was positive for Celiac. Gluten can be inflammatory to the entire body and, especially, the part of the brain that controls balance, integrates with the vestibular system, and helps to inhibit the brain stem. The brain stem is the part of the brain that controls the autonomics. We took her completely off of gluten and, thankfully, her other tests that the neurologist ran including brain scans were all negative for lesions. She completed a 6-month therapy program in our office designed to improve balance and coordination, inhibit the sympathetic nervous system, restore the body's ability to inhibit and gait pain. Her pain level decreased to a zero, balance was restored, memory improved, brain fog lifted and her ability to participate in her normal daily life improved greatly. She continues to perform her exercises at home that focus on the part of the parasympathetic nervous system that calms us down.

Primary Afferent Axons

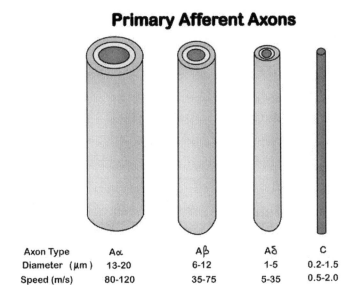

Axon Type	Aα	Aβ	Aδ	C
Diameter (μm)	13-20	6-12	1-5	0.2-1.5
Speed (m/s)	80-120	35-75	5-35	0.5-2.0

CHAPTER FOUR
How Can I Tell If I Have Small Or Large Fiber Neuropathy?

Richard was looking forward to discussing all that he learned with the neurologist as he patiently waited for him to enter the room. He had been reading quite a bit about peripheral neuropathy and was beginning to get a grasp on how complicated this is. He learned a new vocabulary, frankly, one in which he preferred not to.

The doctor began to tell Richard and his wife that he is going to run some tests to confirm the diagnosis and to determine if he has small or large nerve fiber neuropathy.

Finally, some tests, Richard thought. He desperately wanted confirmation that he, in fact, had neuropathy, even though, the descriptions he read were quite accurate in portraying his symptoms.

Small and large nerve fiber neuropathy? More terms?

What Is Small Fiber Neuropathy and Large Fiber Neuropathy?

The two types of nerve fibers we are going to talk about are C fibers, which are small nerve fibers, and A fibers, which are large diameter fibers.

The small nerve fibers or C fibers primarily deal with pain and temperature.

Symptoms of Small Nerve Fiber Neuropathy:

This often begins with a sensation in the feet like you are walking on sand, glass or small pebbles. It can also be described as this sensation of a wrinkle in the sock. There can be symptoms of cold or burning that can vary with activity but generally is worse at night. Since these small nerves deal with pain, there can also be sensations of tingling or a pins and needles sensation.

A classic pattern of the small fiber neuropathy is the stocking and glove paresthesia or a length dependent. However, it can affect the trunk, face and proximal limbs or a non-length dependent pattern fashion.

The most common cause of small fiber neuropathy is diabetes and metabolic syndrome. Research suggests individuals with diabetes and metabolic syndrome have twice the risk of developing neuropathy.

Hyperlipidemia is another major contributor to the development of neuropathy. Hyperlipidemia means your blood has too many fats or lipids in it like triglycerides or cholesterol. It is important to keep triglycerides and cholesterol within a normal range. We want to maintain a good balance of HDL (good cholesterol) to LDL (bad cholesterol).

Other causes of small nerve fiber neuropathy are chronic inflammatory demyelinating polyneuropathy, Guillain-Barre, Celiac Disease, autoimmune diseases such as Lupus and Sjogren's.

How is Small Nerve Fiber Neuropathy Diagnosed?

Most commonly it is diagnosed by history and examination findings. It is very common for the neurological examination to be within normal limits. With testing, there can be more pain with pinprick, or pinwheel testing and a decrease of hot and cold sensation. Keep in mind that C fibers affect pain and temperature.

Skin Biopsy:

The skin biopsy test is becoming increasingly popular, as patients want answers to determine if the small nerve fibers have been affected. This biopsy can examine if the small nerve fibers have been damaged.

EMG and Nerve Conduction Studies:

In small nerve fiber neuropathy, these tests are generally normal. Of course, with neuropathy, there is rarely anything that is clear cut because often times the large nerve fibers will be affected along with the small nerve fibers exhibiting a positive electro-diagnostic study along with a positive skin biopsy test.

Diagnosed With Small Nerve Fiber Neuropathy: Now What?

If the proper testing is performed and the cause of the small nerve fiber can be discovered, there can be overall improvement in symptoms and function.

In clinical practice, we witness this daily, even though, everyone is told that there is no cure. We hope to share what we have learned and guide you to a reduction of symptoms and an increase in function.

Please do not misinterpret this statement. There is no cure or reversal of neuropathy but symptomatic improvement and quality of life can be achieved.

Symptoms of Large Nerve Fiber Neuropathy:

Large fiber nerves primarily deal with proprioception, vibration and joint position sense. They are large myelinated fibers. Myelination is the covering of the nerves which is the insulation that provides effective communication.

Symptoms include numbness and poor balance.

Upon examination, the vibration sense and pinprick are affected and there might be absent reflexes.

Comparison of Large Fiber vs. Small Fiber

Large Fibers

- Weakness
- Muscle Wasting
- Impaired Vibration
- Loss of Position Sense
- Loss of Reflexes
- Positive EMG/NCV

Small Fibers

- Pain
- Autonomic
- Temperature Changes (Burning, Cold)
- Normal Strength
- Normal Reflexes
- Normal NCV/EMG
- Positive Skin Biopsy

Carol had initial complaints of burning in her feet especially when she was in her bed. She experienced some pain in her toes when she walked. Her balance, vibration, muscle strength and reflexes were good. She was hypersensitive to the pinprick and pinwheel. These findings were suggestive of small nerve fiber neuropathy. We implemented a treatment course of infrared light therapy, cold laser therapy, micro-current stimulation, neuromuscular re-education and soft tissue mobilization. Our supplement regimen consisted of nerve and vascular support along with a Ketogenic type diet. Within two weeks, her sensitivity at night improved significantly whereby the burning sensation stopped. She still experienced a slight pain in her toes with walking but following 6 weeks of therapy, this had reduced to a pain level of 2 on an intermittent basis. In fact, she just returned from a two week river cruise without any increase in symptoms.

PART TWO

WHAT IS THE CAUSE?

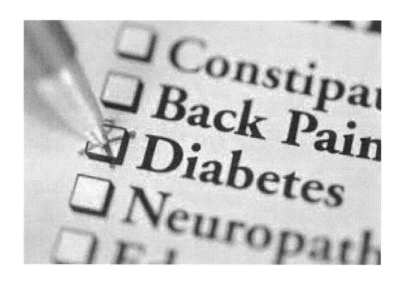

Chapter Five
What Causes Peripheral Neuropathy?

There are numerous causes of peripheral neuropathy, which makes it extremely difficult to identify the origin. They can be acquired, hereditary or idiopathic (unknown origin).
To complicate this further, there are also so many different symptoms and systems that can be affected.

As well, within the medical field, there are so many specialists. Podiatrists for foot pain, neurologists for nerve pain, orthopedists and rheumatologists for joint pain and gastroenterologist for stomach pain. If you are experiencing constipation, vertigo, nausea, cramping in the calves, pain in you feet and tingling in your hands, how many doctors would it take to connect all your symptoms?

Richard began to realize perhaps his neuropathy was occurring years before his symptoms became more pronounced. In the past few years, his primary care doctor prescribed Prilosec for his acid reflux. He saw a physical therapist for plantar fasciitis. His morning routine morning of taking Metamucil to stay regular, and the Ambien at night to help him sleep were perhaps all part of a bigger picture.

He always thought of himself as being healthy and was looking forward to his retirement, but did he and his doctors ignore all the signals? Was this all attributed to just getting older as he was told?

As if all the new terminology was not difficult enough to learn, now they had the task of figuring out what caused this to develop.

Idiopathic Neuropathy? Does that mean they don't know?

His doctor said his blood sugar and cholesterol were good. Now, what?

COMMON CAUSES OF NEUROPATHY

1. Diabetes or Insulin Resistance

2. Lower back problems such as arthritis, stenosis, lumbar disc degeneration or disc herniation.

3. Medications

4. Alcoholism

5. Chronic Inflammation

6. Small vessel disease

7. Cancer/Chemotherapy

8. Poor nutrition or vitamin deficiency (B vitamins and / or D Vitamins).

9. Autoimmune Issues

10. Environmental Toxins

11. Hereditary

12. Cancer

13. Liver and Kidney Disease

IDIOPATHIC NEUROPATHY

It is estimated that idiopathic accounts for 30% of all peripheral neuropathy cases. Essentially, this mean there is no known cause. It has been our clinical experience that most cases of idiopathic neuropathy fall under one of these previously mentioned categories: toxicity, autoimmunity, inflammation and or nutritional deficiencies.

For many of you, the proper tests were never performed to figure out the cause of neuropathy. If you were placed into this category of idiopathic neuropathy, how do you expect to improve without ever finding the cause?

We know that if your neuropathy is caused by lack of B1 and B12 then supplementation or injections should help. We also know that if it was caused by B6 toxicity then we need to eliminate B6 from the multi-vitamins and reduce the foods that have excess amount of B6.

What about the autoimmune issues? Has your Doctor told you how to modulate the autoimmunity so that we can dampen the response to the body? Has the gut-brain axis ever been discussed such as how certain foods or supplements can impact or cause inflammation to the brain which can over time affect the peripheral nervous system?

CURRENT HEALTH CARE MODEL

The healthcare in the United States focuses primarily on acute care. If you suffered from a heart attack, have an acute infection, need surgical intervention, our system is second to none.

However, our current model falls extremely short on the chronic patient. If you suffer from chronic health issues such as peripheral neuropathy, the options for care are limited as well as your chance of improvement.

The approach is to dampen the symptoms with minimal to no emphasis on finding the cause. The testing is designed to determine the type of neuropathy, small or large fiber, but essentially the treatment is the same. Medications!

Medications are prescribed which often create an array of side effects to include brain fog and weight gain. When the initial medications do not work, either the dose is increased, or you are prescribed a new medication.

When the pain gets too severe to manage then a referral to a pain management doctor is executed.

There is no plan for therapy and no hope when the doctor states, "There is no cure for neuropathy."

How can there be a cure if the treatment provided is medications that are designed to suppress symptoms? When I hear these words over and over from my patients, I think how this phrase is so powerful. It makes us not want to try anything that might provide benefit.

In the brief 10 – 15 minute appointments, there is no emphasis placed on the dietary or lifestyle changes that need to take place for a long-term improvement to the current situation.

As previously stated, proper testing is rarely performed to rule out the underlying cause. Tests, which I will discuss later, like a stool sample to evaluate the gut and microbiome; a hair analysis; chemical immune panels; food sensitivity testing to name a few.

To discover the "cause" of the idiopathic neuropathy, a complete set of tests must be performed along with the standard testing of blood work, EMG, NCV and skin biopsy.

Functional Medicine focuses on finding the root cause of the problem. When these are discovered, solutions become much clearer.

Discovering the causes and potential solutions requires a team approach or a doctor that is trained in functional medicine and functional neurology.

Prior to coming to our office, Rocky was evaluated by an orthopedic surgeon, and was told that he would need a knee replacement to relieve him from the pain and the inability to walk without a walker. The difficulty was that Rocky has cerebral palsy which placed an excessive amount of pressure on his knees every time he walked. At 50 years old, he was extremely nervous about a knee replacement and his family shared his concern. Rocky had heard about our clinic and how we had this advanced treatment for knees called cold laser and rapid release therapy. Upon his initial evaluation, I noticed that Rocky was suffering from a form of peripheral neuropathy. It was a compressive neuropathy of the sciatic nerve behind his fibular head, on the outside of his lower leg . This nerve compression was causing a sharp pain in his knee and along the lateral or outside of his leg. Within three treatments, his knee pain had resolved 30 - 40% and after a few weeks of treatment, he cancelled his knee surgery because he had minimal to no pain in his knee. It has been over three years since our treatment program and he continues to do very well and fortunately has avoided the surgery.

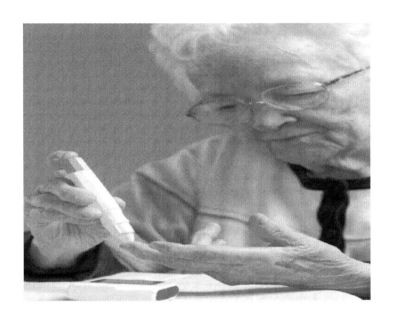

Chapter Six
Diabetic Neuropathy

DIABETIC NEUROPATHY

Diabetic Neuropathy is the most common cause of peripheral neuropathy.

It is well documented within the literature and common knowledge if you have high blood sugar or diabetes, this can lead to neuropathy symptoms. Glucose is our main source of energy. It is transported to all our cells in our body by a hormone called insulin, which is located in the pancreas.

In medicine, all labs that showed fasting blood sugar above 126 is labeled Diabetes. However, nerve tissue is extremely sensitive to values over 100.

When our fasting blood sugar elevates to 100 or above, it is considered insulin resistance. When the cells are bombarded with insulin over a prolonged period due to eating the Standard American Diet (SAD Diet), our cells eventually become resistant to insulin and the glucose accumulates in our body causing our body to store it as fat or triglycerides. The glucose levels in the blood accumulate not allowing our bodies to convert the glucose to the energy we need.

In the early stages of insulin resistance, following a large meal we will find ourselves within a half hour to hour wanting to eat more food. Primarily, this is due to the lack of glucose getting to the cells and converting it to energy.

In the case with Richard, his blood glucose was 101. His doctor did not believe the cause was diabetes but rather labeled him with idiopathic neuropathy.

Another very important marker for diagnosing diabetes is the HbA1c. It is also important to keep the HbA1c below 6.0 but 5.6 or below would be preferable.

Over time, this high glucose becomes quite inflammatory to our body and especially the brain. Approximately, 30% of our energy goes to the brain. If we are not receiving enough glucose, it will begin to affect the communication and the wiring of the nerves by destroying the myelin. It will also impact and begin to damage the small blood vessels affecting blood flow that provides proper nutrition to the tissues.

Diabetes will destroy small and large nerve fibers, typically, small nerve fibers first. There can be burning in the feet in the morning and evening when the hydrostatic pressure of walking is not present. This will create more fluid in the feet which fires off the small nerve fibers and the burning starts.

This is the primary reason why we feel the burning more at night when we get ready to go to bed.

During the day, in the early stages, the small nerve fibers that create pain and temperature are gated or inhibited. However, as the neuropathy progresses and the large nerve fibers become more affected, the feet will begin to burn the entire day and you can experience periodic episodes of numbness.

On a side note, when the small nerve fibers begin to get affected, some men will begin to experience symptoms of erectile dysfunction which was a warning sign that possibly was ignored.

As the neuropathy progresses, it will begin to affect the large diameter fibers that control balance and joint position sense or proprioception. This is not a good sign although the burning might stop, which is always a welcomed relief.

When the large diameter fibers get affected, this will increase the likelihood of falling and performing your normal daily activities without the use of a cane or a walker. The fear of falling becomes so prevalent that you restrict yourself to spending the majority of your time at home on the couch or chair.

In conjunction with the loss of balance is also the progression of the autonomic neuropathy. The autonomics control a lot of functions in the body as we outlined previously. It will ultimately affect the organs as the small vessels bringing nutrients and the nerves have been compromised.

The take home message is to be proactive. You must monitor and control your blood sugar. Diet and lifestyle can reverse type 2 diabetes. The extra effort will be worth the results.

It sounds easy, but making changes are difficult and may require support from family, friends and, of course, your doctor. Please do not just take the medications to control your blood sugar and not make any other changes.

Patterns of Diabetic Neuropathy:

The classic pattern is the "stocking and glove" loss of sensation. This occurs, generally, first in the lower extremities and will progress into the hands.

As it progresses, it can create autonomic dysfunction, vascular changes, and large fiber issues with balance and joint position sense, muscle weakness and atrophy.

Eventually, it can lead to organ problems like kidney disease, problems with the retina in the eye and even necrosis of tissue and potential limb loss.

I have even read where some are calling Alzheimer's, "type 3 diabetes".

Have you ever wondered why when your blood sugar elevates, you would often get confused or had difficulty with memory or a brain fog?

When supporting diabetic neuropathy, it is extremely important to manage food choices. We recommend a Paleo anti-inflammatory type diet or the Ketogenic diet. It does not matter what diet you choose as long as you avoid all processed foods and focus only on whole foods.

High Blood Sugar destroys nerves and vessels.

Healthy Nerves and Blood Vessels

Unmyelinated nerve fiber

Vasa nervorum

Myelinated nerve fiber

Nerves and Blood Vessels Damaged by DPN

Damaged unmyelinated nerve fiber

Occluded vasa nervorum

Damaged myelinated nerve fiber

Since this point is extremely important, I am going to state it clearly so that there is no misunderstanding. If the blood sugar levels are not managed properly, the neuropathy will never improve. The medications that are prescribed might alleviate the symptoms, but the underlying damage will continue.

Ideally, we want our blood sugar between 85 - 100 and the HbA1c below 5.6.

Test your blood sugar regularly and keep it in a healthy range.

As a general guideline, control the blood sugar level by eating small meals throughout the day that includes mostly low glycemic foods to limit the stress on the pancreas and insulin levels. Consequently, there will be less stress on the nerve tissue and a reduction of degeneration.

The glycemic index rates each food on how quickly it influences blood sugar level. High glycemic foods break down quickly and increase blood sugar, like breads, cereals and pastas. On the other hand, low glycemic foods like vegetables cause a steady more sustained release of sugar into the blood. (See Chart of Glycemic Index, Appendix 1)

Eating smaller portions more frequently, grazing on the lower glycemic foods can lead to even better control of blood glucose levels. It is recommended to eat every 2 - 3 hours. We recommend a protein with vegetables and very little starch.

Exercise 20 - 30 minutes a day 5 - 6 days a week has also been proven to lower blood sugar levels.

The ketogenic diet in recent years has gained a lot of traction within the medical community for its benefits for diabetes.

Remember every person is a little different. There might be some that respond better to a Paleo type diet, Mediterranean, or Ketogenic. Discover which will work best for you.

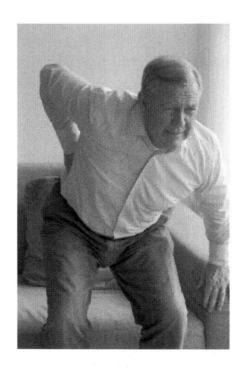

Chapter Seven
Lower Back Pain and Peripheral Neuropathy

The lower back is a very common cause for peripheral neuropathy. The nerves that extend from the vertebral levels L4 - L5 - S1 travel down the leg to the feet. If the nerve flow from this area is interfered with due to a disc bulge, disc herniation or stenosis (narrowing of the vertebral canal), this can cause neuropathy type symptoms.

The disc is a cushion between the vertebrae, which creates ample space for the nerve to travel out of the spinal canal. As we age, this disc, which is hydrated primarily with water, begins to degenerate creating a condition called degenerative disc disease. Consequently, as we lose height in our vertebral motor unit (two vertebrae and a disc), the spinal canal becomes compromised leading to irritation of the nerves as you can see in the illustration below.

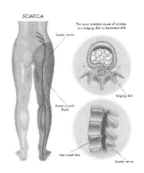

The sciatic nerve happens to come from the lower part of the back and is the thickest nerve in the body. This situation can lead to a compressive type of neuropathy leading to symptoms of numbness, burning, tingling and / or pain.

The neck can be affected just as easily as the lower back exhibiting symptoms in the upper extremity instead of the legs and feet.

This can occur over a long period of time, often without any episodes of lower back pain. However, trauma and / or injuries to the spine and / or disc region will accelerate this degenerative process making the probability greater that some day, neuropathic type symptoms will appear.

Interesting to note that after 30 years of clinical practice, I have seen hundreds of x-rays and MRI's that show degenerative disc disease, stenosis, and herniations without any symptoms. I have come to realize the driving force, once again, behind the symptoms, is inflammation. Once the inflammatory process in reduced throughout the body, we have witnessed time and time again that the patient's symptoms will improve.

To properly diagnose the lower back or neck as a causative factor for neuropathy, a complete evaluation must be performed. This includes a detailed history, an examination including orthopedic and neurological tests. We also recommend diagnostic testing to include x-rays, MRI's, and a nerve conduction study and EMG.

The reliance on MRI's for a diagnosis is all too prevalent these days and the "ART" of a good clinical exam has taken a back seat. In my office, I place more emphasis on the clinical examination and will correlate those finding to any tests the patient might have had.

I guarantee you that a large majority of patients over the age of 65 have some level of disc degeneration and stenosis in the cervical and lumbar spine. It is too convenient to diagnose the cause of neuropathy as this without doing a complete examination.

In many of our neuropathy cases following our examination, if we believe it to be a contributing factor and will also address the spine as part of our treatment protocol.

We incorporate a technique called Spinal Decompression, which has greatly improved our success rate in the treatment of disc issues, spinal stenosis   and neuropathy.

Our spinal decompression treatment is utilized in conjunction with the peripheral neuropathy recovery program. The treatments generally last between 10 - 25 minutes, allowing the disc to rehydrate and absorb important nutrients and oxygen for the nearby blood stream.

It has been documented that the disc space can become increased by as much as 50% by pre and post MRI's.

Post-surgical complications or failures can be another cause of neuropathy. These particular cases are more difficult to treat. In these situations, we endorse a comprehensive approach of reducing inflammation, increasing spinal mobility, strengthening the supportive muscles, providing neurological exercises along with our neuropathy recovery program.

The key is to manage the patient's expectations. Following a failed back surgery, it is unreasonable to believe that you can return to a pre injury level. However, if the daily pain is a 6 and it can be reduced to a 2 or 3, that is a significant improvement.

David had numbness in his feet along with a foot drop. This is a compression of the L4 nerve root causing a weakness of a muscle in the front of the lower leg called the Tibialis Anterior. We ordered a MRI and saw a 7mm disc bulge with compression on the nerve on the left at the level of L4. We began a 3-month course of spinal decompression, peripheral neuropathy recovery program, functional spinal exercises utilizing the vibration platform and TRX. Following 2 months, he had regained the strength of the Tibialis Anterior and his foot drop was gone along with the numbness in his foot. Neurologically, he tested strong to 2-point discrimination, vibration, and motor and sensory testing.

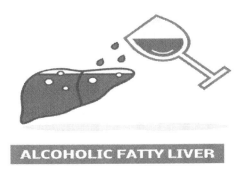

ALCOHOLIC FATTY LIVER

Chapter Eight
Liver and Kidney

The liver and kidney can be a cause of neuropathy due to the body's inability to detoxify leading to high amounts of toxic substances that can destroy nerves.

Alcohol use is the most common type of neuropathy that can affect the liver. Alcohol will also deplete the body's B vitamins, which can also have an adverse effect on the nerves.

There are other causes such as viral or bacterial toxicity that can lead to neuropathy. Hepatitis, Epstein Barr and H. Pylori are amongst the most common causes of infections affecting the liver.

Heavy metal toxicity as well as chemical exposure definitely also needs to be addressed in these cases when it is determined that it is "idiopathic" and the liver or kidney lab markers are not optimum.

Other factors such as genetics and methylation can play a role in overall liver and kidney function.

Kidney or Renal infections or failure can also be a cause of neuropathy. Individuals that are on dialysis commonly have polyneuropathy symptoms.

Lab testing will generally uncover the cause under the guidance of an internal medicine doctor, infectious disease doctor or nephrologist.

In these particular cases, for improvement to occur with the neuropathy symptoms, the cause of the problem must be addressed. For example, if the problem was viral then the proper treatment needs to be employed to reduce or eliminate the viral load.

These neuropathy cases should be co-managed with the appropriate doctor for optimum results.

Depending upon the cause of the neuropathy, we have seen IVIG infusions prove to be successful along with the necessary dietary and nutritional support.

James was an alcoholic for 23 years; although sober now for 4 years, he continues to experience the effects of his addiction on his neuropathy. Alcohol contains high amounts of sugar, which can be very damaging to the brain and nerves. It will also deplete your Vitamin B1, B12, Folate and Zinc, which are important for absorption of nutrients, nerves, detoxification and methylation. James was placed on a specific anti-inflammatory diet, was provided nutrients to support proper nerve growth and function and was put on a liver cleanse. Since his problem was progressing at a very fast rate, we instructed him to do coffee enemas twice per week to support his liver. Along with our nerve activation and nerve recovery program, he began to experience significant improvement during our 6 months. Important to note that his liver enzymes returned to normal and he regained not only the feeling in his feet but, also, his energy during the day.

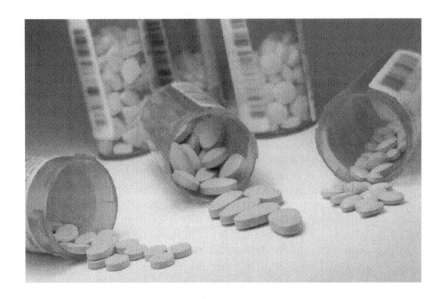

Chapter Nine
Medications

Medications such as statin drugs or chemotherapy has been well documented on how it can contribute to the symptoms of peripheral neuropathy.

However, there are a lot of other medications that have been shown that can cause peripheral neuropathy.

Antibiotics such as Cipro, Levaquin and Avelox are a group of antibiotics called Fluoroquinolone. They are among the most commonly prescribed antibiotics in the United States.

With this class of antibiotics, there are great risks that can come from taking these. Therefore, make sure that when prescribed these that your condition is a serious one and not a minor problem like a UTI or sinus problem.

When I consult with people all over this country, several of the chronically ill have been "floxed"(damaged by the fluoroquinolone). These individuals have had a neurotoxic reaction due to the ability of fluoride to penetrate the blood brain barrier and attack the brain.

Peripheral neuropathy is just one of many problems that can occur due to this toxicity. More common symptoms are tingling, numbness, vertigo, loss of balance, memory issues, tendon ruptures, joint pain, ringing in the ears, rapid heartbeat, intolerance to heat or cold, and rashes.

So, individuals that have been compromised by genetic susceptibilities, MTHFR, methylation, detoxification and the ability to handle chemicals and / or toxins properly get a dose of these fluoride quinolones and this creates an inflammatory state in the body affecting the nervous system, musculoskeletal, gastrointestinal, and autonomic and cardiovascular system.

There is no known cure for Fluoroquinolone toxicity; however, supporting the mitochondria, reducing oxidative stress, reducing brain inflammation, glutathione support and improving the detoxification pathways is a great place to start.

With fluoroquinolones, there can be an immediate reaction and / or a cumulative effect where it will build up in the system and can affect you years down the road. This is why I like to look at genetics and potential susceptibilities to problems that can be changed with diet and lifestyle before they actually occur.

Is it possible that taking Cipro created the peripheral neuropathy or tinnitus years down the road? Is this what idiopathic neuropathy is? Where there is no known identifiable cause, but it is a chemical toxicity caused by an insult to our peripheral nervous system.

OTHER MEDICATIONS THAT CAN CAUSE NEUROPATHY:

Hydralazine (vasodilator) for high blood pressure

Flagyl prescribed for bacterial infections or Rosacea

Macrobid prescribed for urinary tract infections

Dilantin prescribed for seizures

Diana consulted with me after years of struggling with neuropathy due to a reaction to taking her antibiotics. She has struggled with many of the symptoms of neuropathy, burning, numbness, pain, weakness, loss of sleep and depression. An avid cyclist and active person in the past, she found herself at home often times in the wheelchair. We recommended a gluten and dairy free diet, supplements, CBD oil and some exercises to help with her balance and vertigo. Her pain level has decreased. She can now walk without assistance. She has less vertigo and her balance is improving.

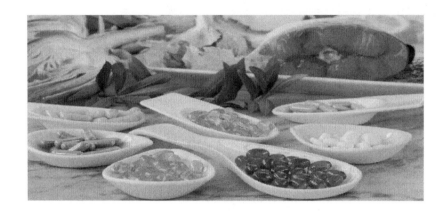

Chapter Ten
Nutrient Deficiencies/Toxicities

Peripheral Neuropathy can be caused by a vitamin deficiency or, at times, even a toxicity as can be in the case of vitamin B6.

The importance of these vitamins and a healthy nervous system or nerve has been well researched. When the nerve is healthy, it allows the sensory and motor nerves to communicate more effectively creating less pain, numbness, tingling and weakness of the muscles.

A healthy nerve consists of a good protective covering called the myelin sheath.

Vitamin B1 (Thiamine)

Vitamin B1 has a lot of functions in the body that are important for the cardiovascular system, brain health, energy production and proper functioning of the muscles in the body. For the nerve cell, it is critical in the development of the protective covering or the myelin sheath. Deficiencies can occur due to excessive alcohol intake, liver and kidney disease and, of course, poor diet. Consuming foods that are processed or have high amounts of sugar can lead to a B1 deficiency.

Vitamin B2 (Riboflavin)

Riboflavin is very important as a behind the scenes role player. There are a lot of functions in the body that require B2 as a cofactor. Cofactors are important pieces to the molecules that actually make them work. The FAD and FMN cofactors require vitamin B2. Most importantly, they allow us to metabolize or break down the food we eat efficiently so that we can turn this into energy. When energy is not produced properly, this will affect the mitochondria of the cell and ultimately impact the threshold to fire the nerve. Signs of B2 deficiency are inflammation of the mouth and tongue. Often times, there will be a cracking at one side or both sides of the mouth, called angular chelates.

Vitamin B3 (Niacin)

Niacin is another important vitamin when talking about chronic health issues and neuropathy. Individuals that tend to have intolerance to cold can be associated with a niacin deficiency. It is essential in the methylation process of the body and, if deficient, people tend to be more of an under-methylator. This can affect energy, neurotransmitters and even sleep. It has been shown to have an impact on brain health, dementia and some psychiatric disorders. William Walsh, PhD has written extensively about this in his book, "The Nutrient Mind". The blood tests are not reliable for B3. Therefore, we generally do not recommend it. We do, however, recommend eating foods that are high in niacin such as the proteins: chicken, beef and fish as well as avocados and nuts.

Vitamin B6 (Pyridoxine)

Vitamin B6 is an essential nutrient that is required for a lot of key functions in the body. Vitamin B6 helps the body make several neurotransmitters which are chemicals that carry signals from one nerve cell to another. Serotonin and Norepinephrine are some of the neurotransmitters that B6 helps to make. It also has an impact on melatonin, which helps regulate the body's internal clock or circadian rhythm. It is necessary for the production of glutathione which is the major antioxidant manufactured in the body. It is also needed for normal brain development and function.

It has been well researched that B6 can help improve neuropathy symptoms. It has also been researched that too much B6 will cause neuropathy. There is a very delicate balance between good and bad levels of B6. My recommendation is to get as much B6 through your diet. Good sources of B6 are vegetables, fruits, whole grains, nuts, seeds and, fish, beef and turkey.

We recommend supplementing only if you have adequately tested your B6 levels. Since B6 is now put into so many vitamins and, even foods and energy drinks, the levels of B6 can creep up on you.

The daily requirement or maximum safe dose is 100 milligrams.

Vitamin B6 deficiency is quite rare and is usually associated with low values of all the B complex vitamins from alcohol abuse, and liver and kidney disease.

Some of the clinical signs would be cracking on the one or both side(s) of the lip, swollen tongue and, depression and confusion.

B6 toxicity is easy to test for through a blood test. If your range is high, it can be a cause of your neuropathy symptoms. By reducing your B6 intake and controlling some foods or drinks that are high in B6, your symptoms should abate.

I do not feel that every neuropathy patient should avoid B6 as it has too many other benefits. As each patient is different, I strongly urge every neuropathy patient to get his or her levels tested prior to beginning any supplement regimen. These should be monitored on a regular basis for many reasons. The obvious reason is to see that your levels are improving. The second reason is to make sure that you are absorbing the supplements and not exceeding the normal ranges.

Vitamin B9 (Folate)

Vitamin B9 is also very important for people with chronic pain and neuropathy. It is necessary in the methylation process to help with detoxification, energy, neurotransmitters, clotting, and the removal of ammonia. It is also required for the synthesis of our DNA.

Dr. Ben Lynch of Seeking Health has educated the public about the importance of folate with regards to the MTHFR gene and its critical role in impacting a lot of the body's major functions and methylation cycle. He has also educated us on the importance of folate as opposed to folic acid, which is synthetic and can cause more harm than good.

Folate is also very important in the prevention of anemia. For every nerve to be healthy, it needs fuel and activation. Fuel is in the source of oxygen and glucose. Therefore, for a healthy neuron to survive, there can be no blood sugar issues or anemias.

Vitamin B12

Vitamin B12 is another essential nutrient. It is, perhaps, the most researched vitamin when it comes to peripheral neuropathy. The reasons are that B12 is important for the health of the nerve that signals the neurotransmitters. It is also important for a healthy myelin sheath that protective covering of the nerve that allows the effective and efficient communication.

Vitamin B12 is also necessary for digestion and absorption as well as cardiovascular health.

These are some of the symptoms that you can experience if deficient in vitamin B12.

- Peripheral Neuropathy
- Chronic Fatigue
- Muscle and Joint Pain
- Poor Memory
- Poor Concentration
- Dizziness
- Depression and / or Anxiety

There are several reasons why your B12 levels might be low.

- Poor Digestion and Absorption
- Vegan Diets
- Medications
- Methylation
- Long term antibiotic use

As we get older, our digestion and ability to absorb the foods can become impaired. This can be due to lack of digestive enzymes or inability to produce enough acid to break the food down properly. Then there is a group of people that have pernicious anemia, which is a condition that their body does not have intrinsic factor, which allows them to absorb B12. This can be seen on a routine blood test called the CBC.

Clinically, we have seen patients consuming a plant-based diet have a deficiency of B12 since animal foods are an excellent source of B12.

Other causes of low levels of B12 that should be addressed by the functional medicine doctor are dietary habits, low stomach acid, called hypochlorhydria, and methylation issues addressing folate and homocysteine.

Some common medications including Metformin and proton pump inhibitors, like Prilosec, also reduce the vitamin B12 levels.

So, when you think about it: your doctor prescribes you a proton pump inhibitor for your acid reflux and metformin to control your diabetes and, ultimately, this can affect your B12 levels and cause nerve damage. The treatment to prevent the diabetes can actually be the source or perpetuating the issue.

We recommend all of our patients over 55 years old to supplement with vitamin B12 as well as our vegan patients.

Excellent food sources of B12 are: Beef, Chicken, Liver, Salmon, Tuna, Turkey, Greek Yogurt and Raw Milk.

The tests I generally run to look at proper nutrient levels are:

- CBC to rule out anemia of B12 or folate deficiency
- Vitamin B12, B1, B6,
- Folate
- Homocysteine
- Methylmalonic Acid
- Magnesium
- Zinc
- Copper

Ethyl consulted with our office and complained of bloating, constipation, and nerve pains in her legs and arms. Her electrodiagnostic testing was normal. Lab tests revealed high RBC, HCT and Hgb. Blood values for B12 were 237. She was a vegan, and had excluded meat and dairy from her diet. After vitamin B12 injections, her levels returned to normal and her neuropathy completely improved.

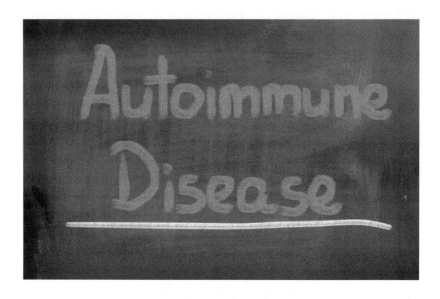

Chapter Eleven
Autoimmune Disease

Autoimmune is a term used to describe a condition when the body's own immune system begins to attack its own tissue. Autoimmunity can be a cause of neuropathy. Sjogren's, Rheumatoid Arthritis and Lupus are some of the more common autoimmune conditions to affect the peripheral nerves.

The cause of some autoimmune conditions is unknown but there generally is a genetic predisposition to the disease. As well, there is a confluence of several factors including a "leaky gut", and some environmental influence or factor that triggers the gene to turn on.

The trigger could be stress, emotional or from trauma. It could also be toxicity from environmental factors like exposure to chemicals, radiation, heavy metals or mold. Food sensitivities, viruses, bacteria, or even parasites could trigger it.

For the purposes of this book and to simplify the process, the immune system is regulated by TH1 and TH2.

The TH1 are the first responders, like the marines in battle. We call them in to fight any bacteria, virus or parasite. They tag the unwelcomed infiltrators, or the antigens. Therefore, our body becomes more efficient at destroying them in the future when exposed.

The TH2 part of our immune system then creates antibodies to help get rid of the antigens.

This TH1 and TH2 part of our immune system is theoretically supposed to be in balance like a teeter-totter. If either system becomes overactive or out of balance, for numerous reasons, this could have devastating effects on the body.

When your body is in a chronic state of inflammation, this means the immune system is stuck in the "on" position. Often, it can lead to the body attacking itself, which is what occurs with an autoimmune disease.

One of the most common areas of the body to fall under attack is the nervous system which leads to symptoms of neuropathy, motor, sensory and or autonomic.

There are a lot of factors that can cause an autoimmune disease and that is why I recommend a functional medicine doctor to explore these   possibilities.

With any autoimmune issue condition, the primary focus is to prevent further destruction of the tissue, as it is not reversible. In doing this, it is important to focus on gut or digestive health since 70 - 80% of your immune system resides in the gut.

Generally, we recommend an autoimmune paleo type diet to eliminate the inflammatory foods and to help heal the "leaky gut". Later in the book, we will discuss in detail about the "leaky gut" protocol we use.

The next focus is on modulating the immune system by prescribing certain supplements to support the Treg cells. These cells help to limit or minimize the immune response.

To enhance Treg cell function, we recommend vitamin D3. Probiotics, omega 3, and tumeric. This is our foundational recommendation and dependent upon what other areas of the body need support, we will layer in some other supplementation.

Julia was diagnosed with Lupus and Hashimotos's which are two autoimmune conditions Her complaints were fatigue, headaches, joint pain, hair loss, and abnormal sensations throughout her body like pins and needles. Electrodiagnostic testing was normal. She was sensitive to pinwheel and pinprick, and had difficulty feeling cool sensations on her feet. She was placed on an autoimmune paleo type diet, prescribed supplements vitamin D, omega 3, probiotics, tumeric, selenium, zinc and alpha lipoic acid. She was in our nerve support program for 3 months. Following this care, her pain levels were greatly reduced. Her headaches and fatigue also improved significantly. We told her about the various stressors that can impact her immune system and instructed her on how to modulate these to minimize future flare ups.

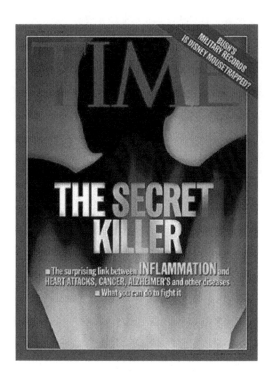

Chapter Twelve
CHRONIC INFLAMMATION AND NEUROPATHY

Chronic inflammation is a very important component in not only causing the peripheral neuropathy, but also advancing and intensifying the problem. There are several factors that cause inflammation and some of them are very much interrelated.

First, it is important to understand that inflammation is a very necessary process that helps our body maintain homeostasis. However, for various reasons, this process can become overburdened and ineffective leading to a chronic state of inflammation.

Inflammation is the common thread that drives most of the chronic health problems we see such as cancer, arthritis, heart disease and neuropathy.

Yet, modern medicine continues to deal with controlling the symptoms of the disease rather than the process, which caused the disease.

There are several lab markers that are useful in measuring inflammation within the body. We look at c-reactive protein (CRP) levels and erythrocyte sedimentation rate (ESR). These are proteins, which can be measured in the blood as the concentrations go up with inflammation.

Some of the more common causes of inflammation can be from a specific or repetitive injury, emotional trauma and chronic stress (who doesn't have that?). Conditions such as anemia, blood sugar issues like diabetes or insulin resistance, and gut health can be causative factors.

When dealing with neuropathy, it is important to look at the entire body, not only the source of injury. For example, if a patient is having thyroid like symptoms such as fatigue, dry skin and their hair is falling out, and a thyroid panel is run and we see a high reverse T3 then we know inflammation can certainly be a part of the cause.

Hormone imbalance can also be a source of major inflammation and stress on the body. Hormone levels should be checked to make sure they are at optimum levels. Do not always give in to the "you are getting old" theory. We all need to become our most informed advocate to help figure out some of the causes.

Liver detoxification issues can contribute to inflammation as the body can have a difficult time breaking down the toxins that we are subjected to on an ongoing basis. If we have continued exposure to chemicals, heavy metals or mold, eventually, the liver will be overburdened and we can see some effects throughout the body. It can manifest itself through skin eruptions, hives, eczema, psoriasis, joint pain, fatigue, neurologically with cognitive decline, or neuropathy.

I personally feel this is the category that contributes to a lot of the idiopathic neuropathy. As I have said before, standard testing does not always show what the issue is. There are labs like Vibrant Health, Doctors Data, Genova Diagnostics, Great Plains Laboratories that are doing great work in helping us identify the cause.

If we just treat the symptoms of burning feet without addressing other pertinent health issues, the success rate or improving the symptoms of neuropathy would not be good.

Drugs like Lyrica and Gabapentin just cover up the symptoms eventually leading to other problems like poor balance, brain fog or weight gain. Initially, there might be some relief. However, since the cause was not addressed, eventually, when you visit the doctor, the dosage will be increased or the medication is changed. Eventually, this leads you down the path of the Pain Management Doctor, depression and continued pain.

I need to be clear. I am not anti-drug or anti medication. In a lot of cases with neuropathy, the medication prescribed will benefit the patient and provide them relief. I am about finding solutions or natural solutions that can achieve the same benefits without all the side effects.

If you do not address the CAUSE of the INFLAMMATION, there will never be a long-term solution.

It is important to maintain a regulatory immune system and support the body's ability to maintain homeostasis and to efficiently deal with the inflammatory process.

How do we control inflammation?

The first place we start with is the factors that we can control such as *diet and lifestyle*. Initially, we eliminate a few foods 100% from the diet. These are gluten, dairy, soy, sugar and alcohol. If the patient has a known autoimmunity such as Lupus, RA, or MS we will also recommend eliminating grains.

These are the most common inflammatory foods and can become extremely toxic to the nervous system and brain.

Next, we provide nutritional support for the inflammation and the Treg cells. The primary support is Vitamin D3, Omega 3, Curcumin, and Probiotics.

There is not one special diet that is perfect for each person. We generally lean towards the Paleo type diets or Ketogenic. Both have been clinically proven to reduce inflammation and improve blood sugar levels.

Lifestyle changes, which we will discuss in another chapter, are designed to decrease stress levels with exercise and meditation. We also discuss with our patients to get quality sleep, breathe properly and maintain proper hygiene.

Common Causes of Inflammation

Candida Sensitivity:

Candida is a fungus in our body that can at times become over abundant, which can create reactions and possible sensitivities. This can occur following a course of antibiotics where the natural flora of the gut is destroyed.

Foods to Avoid if you have symptoms of candida overgrowth are:

- Avoid Sugars: This includes all sweets, cakes, biscuits, anything with added sucrose, fructose, glucose, lactose, honey, maple sugar and cane sugar.
- Avoid Alcohol: This breaks down into sugar

Supplements to be used in conjunction with the anti-fungal diet:

- Garlic: Eating whole or small cloves is best
- Caprylic Acid: This is a fatty acid found in coconut oil which has powerful anti-fungal properties
- Berberine: Found in goldenseal and has strong natural anti-microbial properties.
- Probiotics: Need to restore healthy bacteria with pre- and probiotic formulas.

Gluten Sensitivity:

Gluten and Gliadin are the protein found in grains such as wheat, rye, malt, barley and spelt. We have found this to be the number one inflammatory food and would have our patients remove them from their diet.

Most commonly it is found in bread, pizza, pasta and crackers. Some cereals like wheat bran, shredded wheat and cream of wheat can be an issue and should be avoided.

Some of our alcohols like gin, vodka and whiskey have rye in it which can be reactive and again avoided if you have neuropathy. Beer, which contains barley can be reactive and should also be avoided.

Canned foods, TV dinners and processed meats should also be avoided.

Dairy Sensitivity

The protein found in dairy called casein can be inflammatory and create issues in not only the gut, but also inflammation throughout the body.

It is easy to test for with the elimination diet. Restrict all dairy products for a few weeks and reintroduce them. If your pain is reduced or you are sleeping better and have less brain fog then I would eliminate dairy from your diet.

Not everyone will be reactive to gluten or dairy.

If you have autoimmune issues then I would eliminate them completely from the diet.

Other Causes of Inflammation:

Some of the viruses, bacteria and parasites have become quite efficient in hiding from our immune system. This places the immune system on non-stop high alert. Similar to these insurgents during war, we are always under attack. Our immune system becomes over reactive and hypervigilant in its attempt to find these hidden   foreign invaders.

We have seen conditions like Lyme's and all the co-infections create havoc on our central and peripheral nervous system.

Bacterial issues like H.Pylori or even E. Coli can create inflammatory problems in the body that can lead to immune issues.

Viruses such as Epstein Barr, Hepatitis A, B, and C, HPV Strep, Staph and Herpes Zoster (commonly known as shingles), to name a few, can continue this inflammatory process.

I want to keep emphasizing the importance of a whole body approach to treating or supporting the individual with neuropathy.

There are reasons why you woke up one morning and you had increased sensitivity in your face, arms and legs. Especially when the basic labs are normal and your blood sugar levels are good.

Find the answers and your neuropathy condition will have a better chance of improving.

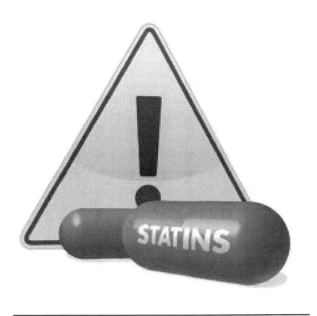

Chapter Thirteen
Statin Drugs and Peripheral Neuropathy

A recent study of a Danish population of 460,000 showed that individuals who took statin drugs were 16 times more likely to develop neuropathy. A similar study of 500,000 people showed that taking cholesterol-lowering medication for one year increased their risk of 15% of developing peripheral neuropathy. After two years of statin drug usage, this number rose to 26%. That equates to 1 out of 4 people taking statin drugs like Lipitor for over 2 years will develop peripheral neuropathy.

The statins can cause an increase in fragility of our cells or early destruction. It can happen to red blood cells, immune cells and nerve cells and the protective covering around the nerve called myelin. Myelin is composed of 80% cholesterol and 20 % protein.

It is not the purpose of this book to discuss the benefits of statins and their effect on reducing the incidence of cardiovascular disease.

It has been argued that cholesterol is not really the problem. It is a response to a problem and that problem again is called INFLAMMATION. When the arterial walls become inflamed cholesterol is called upon the scene to patch or repair the injured and inflamed site. It will do this by closing the vessel wall in a stenosis like fashion.

If your doctor recommends that you take cholesterol lowering statins, it is extremely important that you supplement with CoQ10 (100 - 200 mg). Statins will inhibit the production of CoQ10 and heme. The heme is important for the formation of hemoglobin and myoglobin which are essential for the transfer of oxygen from the bloodstream to other tissues. Oxygen is an important component that drives the production of cellular energy in the mitochondria.

CoQ10 is also important for cellular energy. It is necessary to produce ATP, which is cellular energy. The organ that requires the most amount of energy due to the large number of mitochondria is the heart. Its energy requirements are 200 times higher than skeletal muscle. If you are depleted in COQ10, fatigue and muscle weakness are common symptoms.

Since statin drugs can have a lot of adverse side effects including damage to nerve cells, altered CoQ10 and heme production and an increased risk of blood sugar problems, we recommend different dietary and lifestyle measures to optimize cholesterol.

These are:

- Stop Smoking
- Decrease intake of alcohol
- Decrease sugar intake
- Decrease grains and increase carbohydrate intake from vegetables
- Increase sleep
- Increase Omega 3 fatty acids
- Increase good fats from nuts, seeds and avocadoes
- Increase Saturated fats, (olive, palm and coconut oils)

It is important to note we are not advocating you to get off your cholesterol medications. This should always be a discussion between you and your doctor.

Jack came to our clinic with a burning pain, which he described, "it is like I am wearing stockings." His examination revealed hypersensitivity along the side of the leg with the neurological pinwheel. Jack did not have any prior history of back complaints and / or blood sugar issues. He was, however, on cholesterol lowering medications, statin drugs. Jack began our neuropathy treatment recovery program and was prescribed CoQ10 to counteract the negative effects of the statin drugs. Within eight weeks, Jack's symptoms had improved to the point where he no longer felt the hypersensitivity is his feet or legs.

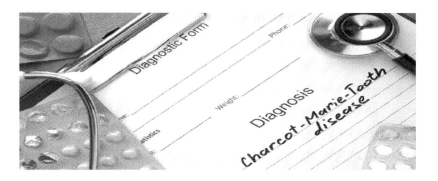

Chapter Fourteen
Hereditary Neuropathy

The most common hereditary neuropathy is Charcot Marie Tooth (CMT), which is estimated to affect 1 in 2500 Americans. Most commonly this occurs in adolescence or early adulthood but can still affect you as an adult. It is a condition that causes the nerves to degenerate and not effectively communicate.

It is diagnosed by physical examination and history along with nerve conduction studies, nerve biopsies and genetic testing. Is there a family history of neuropathy? Do you have high arches and hammer toes?

It affects both motor and sensory nerves. Typically, it can cause weakness of the foot or lower leg causing frequent ankle sprains, foot drop or a high stepped gait.

As the weakness progresses, atrophy of the muscles in the hand can occur making it more difficult to perform normal tasks such as holding a pencil, buttoning clothes or even turning doorknobs.

One can also experience a tingling or burning sensation in the hands or the feet.

If diagnosed with CMT, the strategy is to implement dietary and lifestyle changes. This can have an impact on the progression and help you manage the symptoms better.

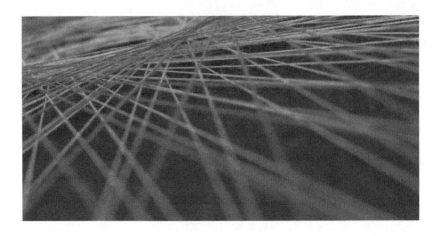

Chapter Fifteen
The Common Thread

As you can see, there are several different causes of neuropathy. It is critical to do PROPER TESTING to identify the UNDERLYING CAUSE.

Clinically, we have seen all chronic health conditions have some common threads.

When I lecture on neuropathy, I always say, "Now, this is the most important part of the entire lecture. Please listen carefully."

"For every chronic condition, there has to be some metabolic imbalance. "

Chronic Health Conditions:

- Peripheral Neuropathy
- Thyroid Condition
- Insulin Resistance

- Diabetes
- Fibromyalgia
- Vertigo
- Sciatica
- Chronic Fatigue Syndrome
- Hypertension
- Chronic Neck/Back Pain
- Stenosis
- IBS
- Insomnia
- Migraine, Chronic Headaches

Metabolic Imbalances:

- Anemia
- Chronic Inflammation
- Unstable Blood Sugar
- Adrenal Gland Dysfunction
- Hormonal Imbalances
- Auto Immune
- Hidden Infections (gut or viral)
- Food Sensitivities
- Medication Side Effects
- Hypoxia, COPD, Sleep Apnea

When there is a metabolic imbalance, it will create a neurological imbalance resulting in a decrease in firing of the brain and nervous system.

Over time if the neurological system is affected, you will notice slight changes in brain endurance. Examples of this are changes in handwriting, difficulty standing for prolonged periods, confusion with directions, memory loss, more sensitive to loud noise and bright lights and sense of smell and taste can be impacted.

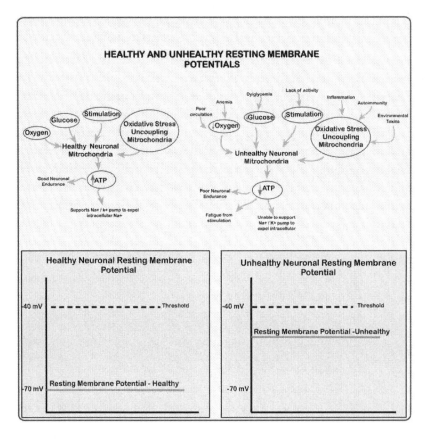

This graph shows the interaction between healthy mitochondria to produce energy and good neuronal endurance. It must include proper oxygen, glucose, stimulation or activation and enough antioxidants to combat the stressors put on the body. In exchange, we have healthy neurons with a good resting membrane potential.

With many factors like anemia affecting the proper oxygen, diabetes affecting the good glucose, a sedentary lifestyle coupled with inflammation resulting from autoimmunity or environmental toxins, this will create an unhealthy mitochondrion. The energy or the ATP of the cell will decline creating fatigue or lethargy and the neuron becomes unhealthier due to the ineffective Na++/K++ pump.

The result is unhealthy mitochondria, poor neuron endurance and the frequency of firing becomes more sensitive. The resting membrane potential becomes more narrowed allowing smaller amounts of stimuli to impact the nerves.

Basically, it requires less activation to get a response. Therefore, we can experience conditions like tinnitus, chronic pain, and fatigue while reading or driving. We can also become more sensitive to the bright lights and loud noise. These are some signs of brain endurance and neuronal health.

My point is don't cover up the symptoms. Instead, discover the underlying cause. This part is not easy. It takes a doctor to not only listen but to perform the necessary tests and examine you properly to make an accurate diagnosis.

Neuropathy symptoms are very difficult to improve if the cause is never found. The nerves will continue to degenerate, and the blood flow continues to become compromised not allowing proper nutrition to the surrounding tissues to heal.

Find the Cause!

PART THREE:

EXAMINATION

AND

TESTING

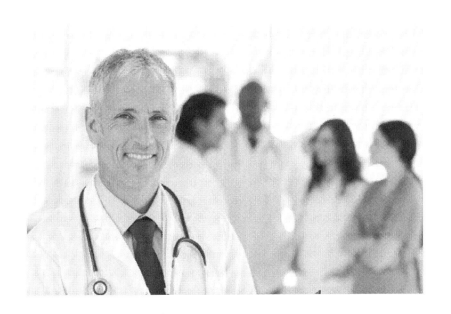

Chapter Sixteen
Testing Performed and Recommended

EXAMINATION AND TESTS

Standard medical evaluation for neuropathy includes a complete physical examination to assess range of motion, muscle strength, and neurological tests such as reflexes, pinwheel and pinprick.

On occasion, electrodiagnostic testing, EMG and NCV might be recommended to measure the electrical activity of the muscles and nerves. This can measure the extent of the damage and, potentially, the cause of the damage.

The goals of the NCV/EMG are to locate the lesion and help determine the type of fiber involved. It can also help determine pathology such as with primary demyelination as in CIDP (What is it?).

An MRI might be utilized to look for nerve compression at the spine and / or periphery that can cause a mononeuropathy type neuropathy.

Blood tests are commonly utilized to check for blood glucose levels, vitamin deficiencies, immune responses and toxicity issues.

This is the recipe used to help the physician in the diagnosis of neuropathy. It appears to be very comprehensive and provides the doctor with an accurate diagnosis.

I guess the question would be why do the majority of patients not improve? In part, because when the diagnosis of neuropathy is provided, regardless if it is small or large fiber neuropathy, primarily the only treatment option is medication.

Commonly, Gabapentin or Lyrica is prescribed to help with the nerve pain. The UNDERLYING CAUSE is not effectively addressed.

Consequently, the symptoms continue, and the dosages continue to be increased eventually leading to more nerve degeneration, fatigue, memory loss and balance issues.

If I were to ask you right now to close your eyes and think of three things that you could do to make yourself healthy?

Would one of those be medication?

The current medical system is proficient at examining a patient, putting them though the necessary tests to confirm the diagnosis but, unfortunately, it lacks the complete whole person approach to treatment. With neuropathy, as we previously discussed, there are many causes which can impact the sensory, motor or autonomic system. It is important to treat the entire person, addressing the cause of inflammation, toxicity, or compression that eventually can lead to a slow degeneration of the nerves.

It is essential when treating neuropathy that we evaluate the patient's entire lifestyle. Physical examination is important, but what led us to this breakdown? Was it the high blood sugar? A vitamin B 12 deficiency? Is it genetic? Are the detoxification and elimination centers of the body, the kidney, liver and bowels functioning properly, getting rid of the waste leading to less inflammation?

All the current treatment is designed to control the symptoms, not the cause. There are neuropathy patients throughout this country searching for answers as their symptoms continue to progress.

If the cause is not addressed, is it not reasonable to think that the symptoms will progress through time causing an increase in the need for medication?

As Richard sat in the examination room, the Neurologist began to perform a thorough exam.

Inspection:

Color:

Initially he inspected the area checking the color. Was there cellulitis? Ischemia? Or Erythema?

Skin:

- Dry/Shiny/Hair loss - peripheral vascular disease
- Eczema/ Hemosiderin staining - Venous Disease
- Ulcers - inspect between toes, on heels and underneath legs

Swelling

- Edema - venous insufficiency/heart failure
- Deep vein thrombosis - tender on palpation

Calluses - may indicate incorrectly fitting shoes or gait abnormality

Deformity Caused by Neuropathy - High arches and hammer toes is a sign of Charcot-Marie-Tooth Neuropathy or Hereditary Neuropathy.

Palpation:

Temperature - cool – Peripheral vascular disease / hot cellulitis

Capillary Refill time - normal = <2 seconds - if prolonged, it may be peripheral vascular disease

Pulses:

- Dorsalis Pedis Artery
- Posterior Tibial Artery- posterior and inferior to medial malleolus

Sensory Examination of the Feet

- Pinprick
- Temperature - laser thermometer
- Vibration Perception (128 Hz tuning fork)

- 1-10 g monofilament pressure perception at the distal halluces

Gait:

- Broad - based- indicative of balance issues
- Foot drop - indicative of L4 nerve root problem

Motor:

- Muscle Strength Testing of Foot and calves

Reflexes:

- Achilles, Patella, Biceps, Triceps and Brachioradialis

LAB TESTS RECOMMENDED

Blood Draw

Complete Metabolic Panel: This will check all electrolytes, liver and kidney functions, and glucose.

CBC with differential: This will check for anemia, infections, possible folate or B12 issues

HbA1c

B1

B2

B6

B9

B12

Folate

Vitamin D

Magnesium

CRP

Homocysteine

ANA

Labs We Might Recommend Finding The Hidden Cause:

Organic Acids Test: This test is one of our favorite tests that frankly most people have never heard of. This test is a nutritional test providing insight into the cellular metabolic process. Genova Diagnostics and Great Plains Laboratories offer this testing.

 a. Intestinal bacterial or yeast overgrowth
 b. Functional vitamin and mineral status
 c. Oxidative damage
 d. Phase 1 and phase 2 detoxification
 e. Functional B complex need
 f. Neurotransmitter metabolites
 g. Mitochondrial Energy Production
 h. Methylation
 i. Lipoic Acid and CoQ10 Status

Hair Analysis: The hair analysis test from doctor's data allows us to see if the neuropathy was caused by heavy metal toxicity.

Glyphosate Testing: Great Plains Lab offers a urine test to look at toxicity levels or the burden of glyphosate exposure. This herbicide is the most common chemical used in pesticides like Roundup worldwide.

Toxic Non-Metal Chemical Profile: Great Plains labs tests for 172 chemicals that we can be exposed to through pharmaceuticals, pesticides, packages, household products, hygiene products and environmental pollution.

Cyrex Labs Offers Several Tests to Figure Out The Cause

Array 2: Intestinal Permeability

Array 3: Wheat/Gluten Reactivity and Autoimmunity

Array 4: Gluten - Associated Cross Reactive Foods

Array 5: Multiple Autoimmune Reactivity screen

Array 7: Neurological Autoimmune Reactivity Screen

Array 10: Multiple Food Immune Reactivity Screen

Array 11: Chemical Immune Reactivity Screen

Array 20: Blood Brain Barrier Permeability

Unfortunately, most of the testing mentioned besides the basic blood work is not covered by insurance. If the patient has been diagnosed with Idiopathic Neuropathy, where there is no apparent cause, we will recommend some of the above listed panels.

Food Sensitivity testing:

Food sensitivity testing or allergy testing can be expensive. We often recommend food elimination and then rotation diet to find the hidden triggers. When your body is sensitive to a food, it can cause an array of symptoms ranging from gastrointestinal symptom, which can be bloating, gas, discomfort and even reflux. They can also create general fatigue, headaches, brain fog and joint pain.

At times the finding out the "why" part of your neuropathy can be quite difficult because it could be a reaction to a chemical they use for flavoring, preserving or coloring.

We recommend beginning with a rotation type diet. It is imperative that you keep track with a food diary and correlate these with your symptoms. The goal is to remove as much processed foods, additives and preservatives as possible.

This step as I said before is the foundational step in improving your chronic pain, illness or neuropathy.

When we eliminate foods that our bodies have become addicted to like sugar, it is possible to go through a bit of a withdrawal symptom. Also, gluten and casein (protein in wheat and dairy) are very addictive to the brain and can create an opioid withdrawal effect. This is due to the peptides from gluten (gliadorphin and casomorphin).

Stool Sample:

Gut infections and bacterial issues are a very common source of inflammation in the body. Infections such as E. Coli, H. Pylori, Clostridia, Candida and Aspergillus can sometimes be the cause of the inflammatory process and the heightened sensitivity. There are labs such as Genova, Vibrant Health, GI MAP and BioHealth that we use.

Electrodiagnostic Testing:

The two most common electrodiagnostic tests for neuropathy are the EMG and Nerve Conduction Velocity Tests. Your neurologist will perform these tests.

They measure the electrical activity of the muscles and nerves and help determine how much nerve damage there is or where the nerve compression is coming from. This will assist the doctor as to outcomes and prognosis with treatment.

Skin Punch Biopsy Test:

The skin punch biopsy is a sensitive and specific test for small nerve fiber neuropathy. It analyzes the nerve fiber density and the damage. Small nerve fibers deal primarily with pain and temperature.

MRI Scans:

MRI scans can allow you to visualize soft tissue lesions. This can include disc herniations, nerve compression, spinal stenosis, and brain pathology.

Jim came to our office with severe complaints of burning pain in his feet especially at night. It became so irritating as he could barely handle the covers touching his feet and / or the feeling of socks on his feet. Following our examination, I told Jim that it was necessary to obtain recent lab work, within 6 months for evaluation. We discovered his liver enzymes were high, his blood sugar was 105 (insulin resistant), and he had a low white blood cell count and a high neutrophil count. This suggests a chronic infection from perhaps a bacterial issue creating inflammation of his liver and affecting his ability to detoxify. We questioned him for alcoholism, but he stated he has not had a drink in over 20 years. I recommended an H. Pylori test which came back positive. He was referred to his primary care doctor for medication to eliminate the bacterial infection which was the driving source of his inflammation. We began a 6-week course of our peripheral neuropathy recovery program and his burning pain was reduced by 85%. He was able to wear socks again and the burning no longer affected his sleep at night.

PART FOUR

TREAT THE PERSON

NOT THE

DISEASE

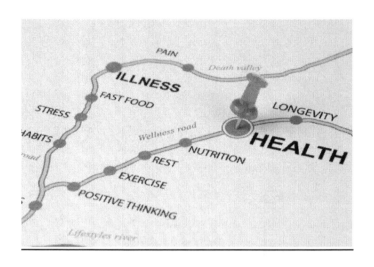

Chapter Seventeen
NEUROPATHY, TREAT THE PERSON, NOT THE DISEASE

For years, I have been telling my patients that neuropathy is one of the most difficult conditions to support and / or treat medically or through alternative methods. In fact, for 25 years of practice, I had no answers for those suffering. I would try different approaches but, in truth, none of them worked consistently. Approximately ten years ago, I began my quest to learn as much as I could to successfully support a patient with neuropathy.

This passion came primarily from watching my father suffer from this. He went from an incredible athlete to being virtually disabled due to his inability to walk without excruciating pain in his legs and feet. He had difficulty walking from his car to the house. I recall the first time I noticed this was when he attended my son's middle school graduation. We had to park less than a block away. After every 5-10 steps, he had to rest just to continue. From that point forward, he just could not attend any of the important functions due to his neuropathy. My Dad was old school and was not going to be seen with a walker or wheel chair. Unfortunately, he spent his last few years sitting in his chair watching TV, hardly the man I remember. It became my passion to figure out how I could help others with the same affliction.

Through years of studying, I learned how to evaluate a person not just from a musculoskeletal viewpoint, which most Chiropractors do but also to incorporate functional medicine and functional neurology. The whole person approach is what we call a Neurometabolic approach. Our success rate with supporting the chronic conditions improved dramatically with this approach.

Through proper testing, we can identify if the problem is coming from the receptor, nerve, spinal cord, cerebellum or cortex. We can identify more accurately if the problem is a metabolic issue arising from inflammation from food intolerances, toxicity, infections, anemia, blood sugar, or autoimmunity.

With an accurate and thorough evaluation, the diagnosis became more precise and the treatment more effective.

In summary, I learned to treat the person, not the disease. Labels are for cans and not for people.

Gary was complaining of phantom leg pain, which he described as an intense burning pain. He had his leg amputated due to complications from his unmanaged diabetes. He recently had a bone scan which showed an infarct of the bone. This means the bone is beginning to die and can be extremely painful. A vascular specialist who said that his circulation was unimpaired also evaluated him. Upon evaluation, we felt that most of his pain was due to a peripheral nerve entrapment along the iliotibial band. This muscle has been associated with the colon according to principles of Applied Kinesiology. We implemented the peripheral neuropathy treatment recovery program and within a few visits, the burning pain had resolved.

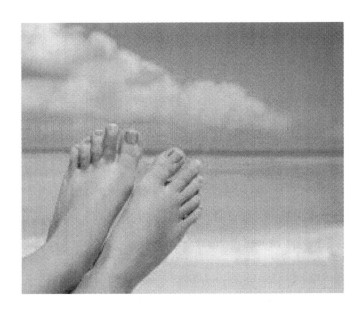

Chapter Eighteen
STRESS AND NEUROPATHY

Stress and Its Effects:

Stress can be physical, emotional or psychological, but often overlap due to several factors such as today's demands and expectations.

Emotional stress can be overwhelming at times and could result from numerous things. With chronic pain and neuropathy, it could be from the fact that since the pain is not visual, many people including our loved ones do not understand the pain and disability that we suffer. This creates an extraordinary amount of burden on relationships with family and friends.

There are also new stresses that now come with social media and how rapidly we are provided information throughout the world. There is not a lot of alone time where we can meditate and enjoy the beautiful silence of nature. Even when we are with someone, rarely are both people present due to distractions of texting, Facebook and television.

Some of the statistics are startling of how many people take anti-anxiety or anti depression medication. For example, 75 million Americans take two prescriptions for anxiety, Xanax and Ativan. It is estimated that one in four women between the ages of 40-50 take antidepressant drugs.

Chronic pain and neuropathy can surely lead to symptoms of depression and anxiety and ongoing stress that need to be addressed.

The first stress we will discuss is that from trauma. This can occur from an accident or injury or a chronic illness. Initially the response of our body is good as it releases a chemical called cortisol to help us manage this stress. However, over time, too much cortisol can become detrimental and have side effects such as fatigue, brain fog and gut symptoms.

The other stress that we are bombarded with, daily, is toxins. Our body can handle quite a bit and it is designed to detoxify and eliminate these chemicals and pollutants that we are exposed to. Sometimes, though, our body can't handle this due to other issues that have burdened our liver, gallbladder, bowels or kidneys. It could be a genetic issue and the inability to methylate properly. What I have found is more and more younger people are experiencing health issues due to this continued onslaught of   toxins and everyday stress.

In the United States, currently there are over 80,000 chemicals registered with the Center for Disease Control and Prevention. These chemicals that are in our air, water, cleaning products, home care products, food preservatives and pesticides may affect our immune system, reproduction system, and hormones.

We even have an internal mechanism to deal with our own toxins the body produces naturally like ammonia, free radicals and carbon dioxide. When these inherent systems do not function properly it becomes increasingly more difficult to get healthy and improve with a chronic illness.

I am sure we all realize how our lifestyle can affect our stress levels. It is important to get proper sleep, preferably 8 hours per day. Exercise at least 20 - 30 minutes every day. Meditation can be helpful as well as prayer. It is also important to eat proper foods that will minimize the toxic burden and lower inflammatory levels. We recommend eating whole foods, avoiding processed foods; even eating organic is beneficial to minimize the amount of pesticides.

Long-term stress as, I mentioned, is not conducive to healing and overall good health because it keeps our body in a heightened state. Our nervous system should be in balance.

We have the sympathetic nervous system, which is more commonly known as "fight or flight." Then we have the parasympathetic nervous system, which can be referred to as "rest and digest. " Now, think about what gets affected with neuropathy and chronic pain. That is correct - rest and digest. We do not sleep well, and we generally have some type of gastrointestinal issues like constipation, diarrhea, acid reflux, food sensitivities or bloating.

While we are under stress it affects the HPA axis. The hypothalamus-pituitary-adrenal axis. This will create potentially a whole array of symptoms or problems as this directly affects hormones and neurotransmitters. Before I get too complicated, the take home message is chronic stress can alter vital hormones, as the body will produce more cortisol.

When an individual suffers from a chronic illness such as Neuropathy, it will affect so many symptoms in the body. It is, in part, why it is so difficult to manage and help relieve some of the symptoms associated with it.

The psychological, physical and toxic parts of the stress is one area that must be managed.

Although, there is no cookie cutter approach to managing stress, we offer a few recommendations.

1. Connect with friends and family
2. Participate in hobbies or activities that you enjoy
3. Listen to music, dance or color
4. Journal every day giving thanks and appreciating what you have
5. Eat an anti-inflammatory diet and avoid sugar, gluten, dairy and alcohol
6. Take adaptogen supplements or herbs to help regulate and manage cortisol
7. Meditate
8. Supplement with Probiotics, vitamin D, turmeric and omega 3
9. Minimize exposure to environmental toxins
10. Join support groups such as the "**Chronic Pain: Understanding, Managing and Improving Neuropathy and Fibromyalgia**" on Facebook. This is a group I created and am the administrator for.

11. Get Professional Help if symptoms become too difficult to self-manage

Sam entered our clinic with complaints of numbness and burning in his feet and up past his ankles. He described the sensation like he was wearing socks. Following a comprehensive neurological, orthopedic and metabolic evaluations, Sam had a very high glucose level for which he was taking metformin. Unfortunately, his glucose was at a level that it was damaging peripheral nerves. Complicating the treatment was the fact that Sam had sciatica pain stemming from a bulging disc in his lower back. Sam agreed to the diet and lifestyle changes and began our spinal decompression and peripheral neuropathy recovery program. Within a month his symptoms were reduced from a pain level 7 to a 2.

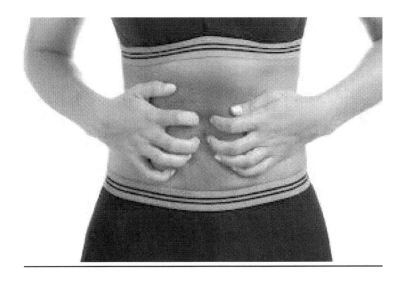

Chapter Nineteen
Why the Gut

With our neuropathy patients, the first area we address is the gut. By gut, we mean your digestive tract, the stomach, small and large intestine, and gall bladder. It is imperative that the gut functions at an optimum level for the simple fact that 70-80% of your immune system resides in your gut. If the gut is unhealthy for a variety of reasons, the body will have a difficult time addressing the inflammation and / or immune response.

The most common reason we see clinically is food sensitivities that over time create an inflammatory response. Eventually, this will affect the tightly woven network of cells that prevent the invasion of viruses, bad bacteria, parasites and large undigested food particles. The tight junctions in the gut become more permeable allowing these invaders into the bloodstream further irritating your immune system. We call this leaky gut syndrome.

All those times when you thought you must have eaten a bad meal because your stomach was upset or created acid reflux, were probably signs of a leaky gut syndrome.

LEAKY GUT

It has been shown that chronic inflammation of the gut from food sensitivities such as gluten or dairy, chronic blood sugar issues or chronic stress can lead to damage inside the lining of the digestive tract.

Proteins that should be absorbed into the digestive tract can leak into the bloodstream creating inflammation throughout the body. The villi of the lining and the tight junctions that hold the gut together become affected allowing these proteins to circulate.

Once again, it is imperative that if you have neuropathy, you must get checked for leaky gut and gluten sensitivity. If gluten sensitivity is a reason you have neuropathy, your current treatment plan will not be as successful or more than likely fail. You MUST get the proper tests done to see if you are reacting to gluten, if you have antibodies (autoimmunity) or if you are genetically predisposed to gluten sensitivity.

The other extremely important component is the inside lining of the digestive tract must be healed and sealed. In our clinic, we use several products along with an anti-inflammatory diet to accomplish this.

We have a lot of patients that come to our clinic and explain that they went gluten free and saw no change in their symptoms. There are a few reasons for this.

First, they were not 100% compliant in the elimination of all gluten from their diet. If you have gluten sensitivity and a leaky gut, it must be 100%. They must eliminate all gluten grains like wheat, rye, and barley. However, that is only the first part.

The other component is and, unfortunately, this is what makes neuropathy and chronic health conditions difficult to treat, is that it is not always just gluten. It could be dairy, soy, or a host of other foods that can create these issues.

There are no two people that are the same, so we recommend a complete removal of all wheat, dairy, soy, sugar and alcohol for a minimum of 3 weeks. At that time, slowly introduce one at a time to determine which one you are sensitive to, if any. This is a lot cheaper than spending money on testing and virtually you can have your answers within a few weeks.

The shotgun approach where you try one thing generally will not work. That is why when you have purchased the special cream or supplement, it never works.

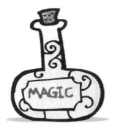

I stated numerous times in this book the most prepared individual to develop this plan is one who is well versed in Functional Medicine and Functional Neurology. I, also, am in favor of a team approach where a Neurologist works closely with and Internal Medicine Doctor and a Nutritionist to develop a clear treatment plan.

With regards to our comprehensive plan for gut health, we adhere to the 4 R program - *Remove, Repair, Replace and Rejuvenate.*

That is *Remove* the bad bacteria, fungus, parasites, and foods that are creating the stomach irritation. We use a combination of herbs and supplements to accomplish this.

The second critical component in the reduction of inflammation and a decrease in symptoms, is the digestive lining must be *Repaired.* The lining is extremely irritated from the years of eating gluten, grains, processed foods and sugar. Products like glutamine, licorice root, aloe, ginger and colostrum help to repair the gut lining.

The third part of our program is the *Replace* phase. The digestive system is exposed to a lot of various bacteria, parasites and has an innate ability to remove these foreign invaders. However, when the body is exposed to inflammation for prolonged periods, these invaders become more prevalent and take advantage of an unhealthy situation. We use probiotics and, occasionally, other products, to replace the bad bacteria with good healthy bacteria.

So, the plan seems simple. Eliminate the foods that create the inflammatory process, heal the digestive lining and replace it with good bacteria that allow us to fight better.

Rejuvenate is the last phase. We want to make sure we have good digestive enzymes to digest our foods, proper B12 levels for absorption, proper acid in the stomach and good Vagus Nerve Stimulation to keep the process functioning well.

There is a brain-gut axis as well as gut-brain axis. What affects the gut will, in turn, affect the brain and vice versa. The brain fog that you can be experiencing might, in fact, be an issue with the digestive system.

The brain, like the gut, has a barrier that should not be permeable. However, sometimes these foreign invaders cross the blood brain barrier and create a cytokine or inflammatory reaction in the microglial cells. This can create a wide variety of symptoms to include balance problems, headaches, high blood pressure, constipation, tinnitus, and even depression and anxiety.

The Vagus nerve is our rest and digest nerve. If functioning properly, it will maintain proper secretion of acid to help digestion and motility.

If you are constantly stressed, have difficulty sleeping and suffer from constipation, you can have some Vagal Nerve issues.

We recommend employing simple techniques to stimulate the Vagus Nerve such as belly breathing, gargling, humming or stimulating the gag reflex.

In the beginning, these diet and lifestyle changes appear daunting. However, once you adapt and your symptoms begin to disappear, including some you did not know were related such as energy levels and better sleeping patterns to name a few, you will have a choice. The choice is clear, eat an anti-inflammatory diet and feel better or don't.

It is imperative that following the elimination of certain foods, upon reintroduction, to identify the foods responsible for this inflammatory response and remove them from the diet. Some of them will need to be removed permanently. I recommend writing them down as it is easy to forget.

To summarize, the gut must be healed to have an accurate and beneficial immune response. We utilize not only dietary measures to reduce the inflammation in the body, but certain supplements to help support the tight junctions to allow the tissue to heal.

Also, dependent on the complete analysis of your lab work, we might suggest further testing to uncover the hidden cause or infection.

The detective work is the essential component in supporting

 patients with neuropathy.

Gloria came to our clinic with complaints of knee, hand, ankle and foot pain due to her Rheumatoid Arthritis. Following evaluation of her labs and a thorough examination, we placed her on an anti-inflammatory diet and recommended supplements to support the leaky gut and regulate her immune system. She began the peripheral neuropathy recovery treatment program along with cold laser and within 3 weeks, her pain level went from a 7 to a 3.

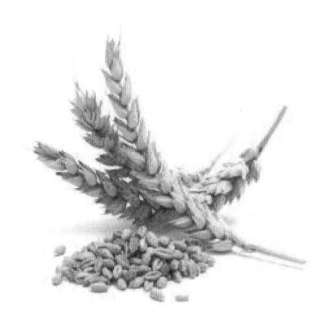

Chapter Twenty
GLUTEN FREE: IS IT A FAD?

In 2002, the New England Journal of Medicine listed 55 "diseases" that can be caused by eating gluten.

Gluten (from Latin *gluten*, "glue") is a protein composite found in foods processed from wheat and related grain species, including barley and rye. It gives elasticity to dough, helping it to rise and to keep its shape, and often gives the final product a chewy texture. Gluten may also be found in some cosmetics or dermatological preparations. While we have all been told that whole grains are good for us, nothing could be further from the truth if you have gluten sensitivity.

The number of people that have sensitivity to gluten is on the rise and the effects of gluten on their bodies can be devastating.

Gluten sensitivity creates inflammation throughout the body and can lead an autoimmune (your immune system is attacking your own body) disease, with wide-ranging effects. It can affect the skin, nervous system and / or the digestive tract.

Often, the symptoms of gluten sensitivity are silent in the gut. The individual will be unaware that they have a problem until it manifests itself in the gut, skin, brain, peripheral nerves or extraspinal regions to include other joints in the body.

I am often asked why suddenly has gluten become such an issue in people? First, it is very difficult to find "pure wheat" in this country. Wheat has gone through a hybridization process and some people feel that we have difficulty digesting this new form of wheat. Our bodies interpret this as a foreign protein.

The other reason why gluten has become the leading food sensitivity that I have seen in recent years is called deamidation. To allow the gluten to become more soluble in water, they perform an enzymatic process called deamidation. This allows the gluten to become more soluble and can be used as filler in many of our foods and cosmetics.

Neuropathy can occur over time when this unrecognized food sensitivity has created a state of inflammation in the body. For the individual suffering from this neuropathy, you could see how difficult it would be to attribute the burning pain in their feet to the stomach and/or gluten sensitivity. However, as more research is being done, it is proven to be a driving force behind the inflammatory process, autoimmune disorder and in turn peripheral neuropathy.

The role of the health care practitioner is to treat the whole patient and be a detective to discover the cause of the inflammatory process. This often requires special testing. Besides the standard blood chemistry panels, we utilize Cyrex Labs. Presently, this is the gold standard in testing for gluten sensitivity. It checks for 11 different types of gluten. The test will also tell you if you have antibodies present affecting the skin, nervous system or gut.

The gold standard in the medical community is the Celiac Test. For this to be positive for Celiac disease, a patient must have a biopsy that shows tissue destruction in the gut as well as the gene mutation HLDQ2 or HLDQ8.

It is extremely important to always perform the proper testing which sometimes means digging a little deeper than the standard metabolic panel and CBC.

If you have the genes for gluten sensitivity and you grew up eating gluten, it is just a matter of time until you have insulted your immune system, enough that it will respond by creating an autoimmune disease or Celiac Disease. There are many different autoimmune diseases that are possible, but in this chapter, we will focus on neuropathy.

Every time a gluten sensitive person eats gluten, it will spark the immune system into action. Gluten is perceived as an invader from the outside that does not belong in our body, just like bacteria and viruses. Antibodies are produced against gluten so that the next time you eat it, the immune system is even more efficient at mounting an attack. The problem lies in the fact that the same antibodies, the GAD65 antibodies, affect many body tissues, like the cerebellum in the brain and pancreas.   The pancreas is where insulin is produced and the cerebellum is the balance center of the brain.

Gluten in molecular structure, is also very similar to certain tissues in the body like the Thyroid. As these proteins circulate your body, they will attach to tissues that has a similar molecular structure. However, the organ recognizes it as an outside invader and, thus, they begin to fall under attack from our own immune system. This is what is called molecular mimicry and is common in Hashimoto's Thyroiditis. This, of course, is an oversimplification of an autoimmune disease and the process, but I think it will help you get the picture.

In the Journal of Neurosurgical Psychiatry in November of 2006, there was an article about Neuropathy associated with gluten sensitivity. The conclusion was "gluten sensitivity may be etiologically linked to a number of idiopathic axonal neuropathies."

There is that word "idiopathic", again. It means unknown cause.

Ellen came to our clinic with complaints of widespread joint pain and a tingling sensation in her hands and feet. Upon examination, it was noted that she had skin irritation and rashes on various parts of her body. We ordered the Cyrex 2, 3 and 4 arrays. Cyrex 2 exhibited she had a leaky gut and her intestinal membrane was more permeable. Cyrex 3 showed she had gluten sensitivity to 6 different types of gluten. Cyrex 4, which tests for 18 foods that cross-react with gluten, revealed that she cross-reacted with rice and chocolate. We removed the reactive forms of gluten and cross-reactive foods and implemented our intestinal repair and neuropathy recovery program. Within two weeks, the joint pain had resolved. She was sleeping better and had more energy. Following six weeks, her rashes were all but gone. Ellen over the past year has realized when she eats certain types of foods, her body will react, and the skin will become more sensitive, and all of her joints will ache. For the moments when she is going to a party or be in a situation where she cannot control her food intake, she will take the supplement we recommended to abate her symptoms.

PART FIVE

TREATMENT

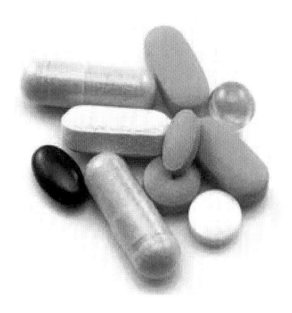

Chapter Twenty One
Supplementation and Neuropathy

There is a lot of research on supplements and how they support healthy nerves and blood vessels. Let me be clear: there is not one program that will benefit each one of you. I also will tell you not to buy into the hype that is presented by all the magic pills out there that, theoretically, is going to cure your neuropathy.

The following recommendations are based on research and it is a comprehensive program designed to support the body. Therefore, it can begin to heal itself.

We recommend using high quality supplements because some of the cheaper vitamins have unwanted excipients that are probably not the healthiest for the cell and our goal is recovery.

We discussed earlier some of the tests and deficiencies or toxicities associated with these such as vitamin B12, B1, B2, B6, Folate and D. Get tested and see your values prior to starting any regimen.

There is some question as to whether or not high vitamin B12 levels are good for you? I am not sure if I have the correct answer, but in my opinion, and within the Functional Medicine community when values are high, we interpret this is as a malabsorption problem with Vitamin B12 or potential receptor resistance.

I do not think there are any dangers with high levels of B12 except that it might not be working as well as you think it is.

Prior to starting any supplement regimen, make sure you discuss this with your doctor to make sure that there are no contraindications with any medical condition you might have or potential drug interactions.

These are general recommendations that I use to support the majority of my patients.

SUPPLEMENT RECOMMENDATIONS:

FUNDAMENTAL SUPPORT

- **Vitamin B12**- I personally like a combination of adenosyl / hydroxyl B12 with methylcobalamin. If the combination is difficult to find, go with the methylcobalamin. The best form of delivery is sublingual or liposomal. I personally prefer the liposomal but it is a bit more expensive. Try to avoid the Cyanocobalamin.

- **Omega 3 Fish Oil** - I recommend approximately 2 grams of a combined EPA and DHA. If you are having brain fog, fatigue or memory issues, focus on higher amounts of DHA. Fish oil is excellent for many reasons including reducing inflammation, overall brain function and cellular toxicity. Nordic Naturals is well known for their high-quality Omega 3. This is one of those supplements where it is necessary to get high quality due to the potential of the fish oil becoming rancid and doing more harm than good in the body. Some good natural sources of omega 3's are from salmon, mackerel, flaxseed, walnuts and dark green leafy vegetables.

- **D3** - Your Vitamin D levels ideally should be around 50-70. Commonly, people are deficient. Therefore, we recommend 5000 IU per day. If your labs suggest that you are extremely deficient then talk to your doctor about prescribing high dose of vitamin D, at 50,000 IU. Vitamin D3 is important for nerve growth and function. It is also important for immune health. There are a lot of companies that sell a high- quality Vitamin D. Generally, I like to include it with K2 to help with calcium absorption for proper bone health. Vitamin K2 is not for everyone due to clotting issues. Therefore, make sure you consult with your doctor.

- **Probiotic** - Probiotics are living microorganisms that when ingested, provide many health benefits. I recommend changing brands every 3-4 months, so that we do not mono colonize the same bacteria. They are also best taken at nighttime before bed. The most common probiotic bacteria include Lactobacillus, Bifidobacterium and Saccharomyces Boulardii.

- **Magnesium** - Magnesium glycinate or chelated magnesium is recommended at 200 mg.

- **Curcumin** -This has potent anti-inflammatory affects. Too much inflammation can interfere with optimum blood flow. We recommend 500 mg once daily with food.

MITOCHONDRIAL SUPPORT:

- **Alpha Lipoic Acid** - We recommend R-ALA because it is the natural form and not the synthetic. It is recommended for diabetic neuropathy and patients that suffer from burning and numbness. It is also beneficial for nerve repair.

- **COQ10** - 100-200 mg per day. Good antioxidant and beneficial for mitochondrial health. Statin drugs deplete enzyme to make COQ10. Therefore, make sure you supplement.

- **Acetyl L Carnitine** - Recommended 350-500 mg twice per day. Acetyl L Carnitine helps to convert fat to energy along with Magnesium. It is also good for brain health and cognition.

GUT HEALTH

- **REPAIR**: To repair the gut lining, we use a combination of products in specific formulas. L-Glutamine, Slippery Elm, DGL, and Aloe Vera. Theses product have proven to be effective to seal the border and heal the leaky gut.

- **REMOVE:** Bacteria, Fungus and Parasites need to be removed. Anti-bacterial supplements to assist with this are Oregano Oil, Berberine, Garlic and Pau d'arco. Anti-Fungal herbs are Caprylic Acid, Tea Tree Oil and Coconut Oil. Anti-parasitic supplements include Wormwood, Black Walnut and Grapefruit Seed Extract.

- **REPLACE:** We replace with probiotics taken before bed and switch brands every 3-4 months.

- **REJUVENATE:** - Digestive enzymes are necessary to help us reduce inflammation in our gut, improve digestion of food and helps us assimilate nutrients. It is also beneficial to reduce food sensitivities and reduce risk of autoimmunity. We also like to add Taurine and Ox Bile to assist with the bile salts and the digestion and absorption of fats.

LIVER DETOXIFICATION

We are bombarded by toxicity every day. They are in the foods we eat, the air we breathe, the water we drink and the cosmetics we put on. Our liver is designed to handle these toxins and make them water soluble so that we can eliminate them properly. The liver should be supported on a daily basis.

- **NAC-** 500 mg 1 -2 times per day.
- **Milk Thistle/Silymarin**

- **Glutathione -** I prefer a liposomal form.

DIABETIC NEUROPATHY

- **Metabolic Synergy -** This formula from Designs For Health is a good multivitamin/mineral that is beneficial for the glucose metabolism and insulin receptor sites.
- **Fundamental Support -** This is the B12, Fish Oil, D3 and probiotic I recommended above.
- **Acetyl L Carnitine -** Recommended for brain health and overall energy. Helps transport fatty acids.
- **Alpha Lipoic Acid -** R-ALA. Seeking Health and Life Extension has R-ALA.
- **Inositol -** Inositol assists with the function of Alpha Lipoic Acid
- **NOx Synergy -** Optimizes Nitric oxide levels in the body. This helps vasodilation and promotes healthy microcirculation.
- **Citrulline -** Has also proven to be very effective with nitric oxide levels

BRAIN FUNCTION AND REPAIR

- **COQ10 100 –** 200 mg is a powerful antioxidant and, also, a cofactor for the creation of ATP, the energy in every cell.
- **Fish Oil -** DHA in particular is the omega 3 fatty acid that is responsible for brain function and repair.
- **Probiotics -** Simply put healthy gut = healthy brain. Keep the gut flora healthy to maintain its ability to function and absorb nutrients.
- **Curcumin -** Anti-inflammatory.

- **Flavonoids** - Provide protection and anti-oxidant support for the brain. Luteolin, Catechin, Apigenin, Rutin.

CIRCULATION:

- **Omega 3 fatty acids**
- **L-Arginine** - Helps to expand blood vessels, reduce blood pressure and improve circulation. Dosage 1000 mg one or two times per day.
- **Curcumin** - This anti-inflammatory will improve circulation. Recommended dosage 500 mg once per day with food.
- **Niacin** - This has been proven to improve circulation in the extremities. Recommended dose is 1200 mg daily of niacin.
- **Vitamin C and Bioflavonoids** - Support healthy blood vessel function, microcirculation, capillary flow and vascular tone.

In our office, every patient is provided a supplement regimen that is specific for their condition to lower the inflammatory levels and support the tissues or organs that are not functioning properly.

THERE IS NOT ONE PROTOCOL THAT WILL BENEFIT ALL TYPES OF NEUROPATHY.

It should be apparent that there are way too many causes and types of neuropathy to receive benefit from one supplement or one protocol that is supposed to benefit everyone.

Supplements are designed to do just that. Supplement the food that you are eating. In my opinion, the dietary and lifestyle choices you choose will have a greater impact on your overall health than any supplement program.

The goal is to identify the cause and help to support the weakness. These recommendations are also suggestions and should not be construed as medical advice. Prior to taking any supplement, you should consult with your doctor to make sure there are no contraindications with the medications you are currently taking.

Please purchase high quality supplements to avoid excipients and unwanted chemicals or substances in your vitamins. We certainly do not want these going to the cell along with the good nutrients we need.

On our Facebook Support Group, we will be discussing supplements, herbs and brands. The group is **Chronic Pain: Understanding, Managing and Improving Neuropathy and Fibromyalgia.**

Once again, these are recommendations only from what I have researched and seen clinically. With Neuropathy, there is no one size that fits all. An accurate diagnostic supportive plan must be assembled following a thorough history, review of labs and examination.

I have enclosed research to support the various recommendations, but please do your own research, coordinate it with your labs and discuss all choices with your doctor.

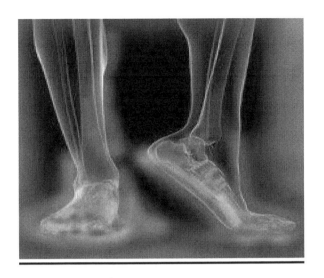

Chapter Twenty Two
Pain Support

NEED RELIEF: TRY THIS

Cramping:
- Epsom Salt bath
- Electrolyte Foods: yogurt, bananas, watermelon, avocado and coconut oil, pickle juice
- Hylands Leg Cramps (OTC)

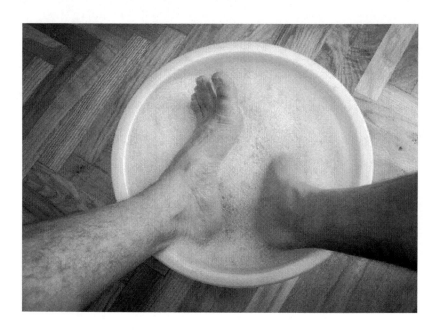

Nerve Pain/Burning:
- Magnesium Lotion by Life-Flo. Massage onto hands and feet.
- CBD oil if legal in your state.
- Take supplements to improve microcirculation. Bioflavonoids, Gingko Biloba, Horse Chestnut can be beneficial.

Muscle Tightness:
- Roll calves and feet with massage stick.
- Use hand held vibrator on calves and feet.

Balance Issues:
- Avoid gluten, dairy, alcohol.
- Practice balance exercises every day to improve.

Cold Feet:
- Soak in warm water or take warm shower.
- Increase circulation in feet with exercises to lower extremity.
- Supplement with flavonoids and arginine.
- Infrared or cold laser therapy to improve circulation.

Pain Relief:

- **Electric Stimulation:** Electric stimulation in the form of H-wave therapy like the Hako-Med; Micro-Current, TENS machine or Rebuilder. Be careful with neuropathies from Complex Regional Pain Syndrome and Post Stroke since electric stimulation and vibration can exacerbate symptoms.

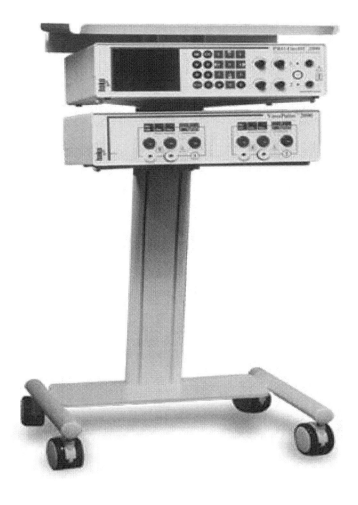

- **Infra Red Therapy** - Infrared therapy assists with the release of nitric oxide. Nitric oxide enhances blood.

flow and brings nutrients to the tissues to help them heal.

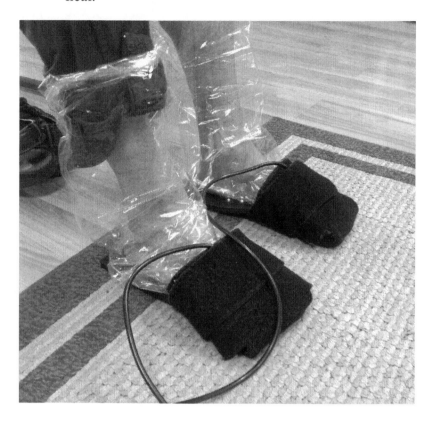

- **Cold Laser Therapy** - Cold laser enhances microcirculation which increases blood flood. It is beneficial in treating the underlying causes of neuropathy.
- **Pulsed Electromagnetic Therapy** - PEMF has been proven to be beneficial in reducing neuropathic pain as well as improvement in nerve conduction.
- **Vibration Therapy** - Whole body vibration was found to reduce the pain from diabetic neuropathy. We use this type of therapy in our office with every neuropathy patient.

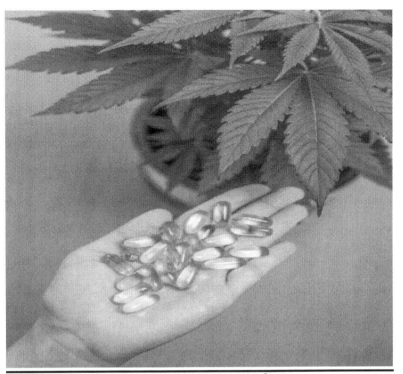

Chapter Twenty Three
CBD OIL: MEDICATION ALTERNATIVE

Cannabinoids are the primary compound produced by the cannabis plant. There are currently over 110 cannabinoids that have been discovered. The most common come from marijuana and hemp.

CBD or cannabidiol is a non-psychoactive cannabinoid that is found in the hemp plant. Hemp is the largest producer of CBD with low amount of THC which is the psychoactive ingredient in marijuana. In essence, with CBD, because of the low amount of THC, you will not get that "high" feeling. All hemp products contain less than .3% THC. This is the acceptable limit to ship THC across state lines legally.

In the last 20 years, researchers have discovered a natural cannabinoid receptor system in the human body. These receptors CB1 are found primarily in the brain, spinal cord and certain peripheral tissues. The other receptor CB2 has been proven to boost the immune system.

CBD is proven to be a great natural anti-inflammatory agent. There are a lot of research papers that confirm the effectiveness of CBD oil and chronic pain. In 2008, a review was conducted looking at all the studies between the late 1980's and 2007. They concluded that CBD was effective in pain management without any adverse side effects.

It is important that you also work on the dietary and lifestyle changes discussed in this book along with the CBD oil to have the greatest impact on your pain levels.

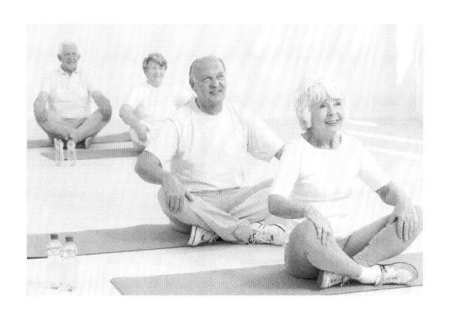

Chapter Twenty Four
Peripheral Neuropathy and Exercise

Exercise is an essential component of the peripheral neuropathy recovery program. When a patient comes to our clinic, generally, their neuropathy symptoms have gone on for quite some time and they have an overwhelming fear of losing their balance and / or falling. Their lives have become sedentary since sitting in their chair eliminates, temporarily, this fear. So, the cycle begins, the more they sit, the more deconditioned they become which increases the propensity to fall.

It is not uncommon for people that suffer with neuropathy to get frustrated when the doctor tells them to exercise given the fact that, sometimes, it is hard enough to walk from the bedroom to the bathroom.

Everyone should be assessed on the ability to exercise and general strength and fitness level. Then various exercises are prescribed to facilitate movement and to improve function.

For all nerves to heal and function properly, they require fuel and activation. Fuel is in the form of proper glucose and oxygen and activation is stimulation, which can occur during exercise.

We are all aware of the benefits exercise is for our cardiovascular system, but it is equally important for proper function of the brain and nerves.

Which exercise is the best?

The best exercise simply stated is the one you are going to do or that you can perform. For example, if you are having difficulty with your feet which eliminates walking then some alternatives could be bicycling or swimming. Some cities have pool therapy for seniors and arthritis sufferers where they keep the water temperature warm and do a gentle low impact water aerobics work-out.

Resistance bands or light-weights are another good form of exercise if you are having difficulty walking.

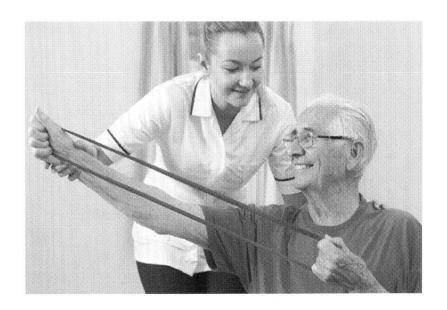

With any exercise regimen, there will be a few challenges. The first challenge is: am I able to even perform the prescribed exercise. In the beginning, tailor the exercise to what you can do. If you have difficult with walking and are in a wheel chair then begin with upper extremity exercises.

The second challenge is getting into the routine. New habits are difficult to start especially when results are not seen immediately. Set reminders, which can be timers, post it notes, and take the initial step and begin.

The third challenge is becoming creative to incorporate all body parts. There is a lot of information now online about various chair exercises or chair yoga that will provide ideas to make it suitable for you and your condition.

Remember the best exercise is the one that you are going to do. I also know for a fact that if you become more sedentary and do not provide adequate circulation to the muscles and nerves, they will continue to deteriorate.

Why It Is Worth It

Exercise is important to maintain strength, increase circulation, improve balance and coordination and allows us to live independently. It has been proven to reduce heart disease, lower blood pressure, lower blood sugar, improve insulin resistance, reduce risk of developing Alzheimer's and strengthen bones.

My two biggest fears as I age are falling and dementia. Exercise helps with minimizing my risk for falls, and developing memory loss.

Our entire life, we have paid for various insurances for protection against certain situations, accidents, fires, earthquakes, disability, and health. We have spent a lot of money over the years for this security and protection. However, our most important investment, our health, sometimes falls short. The good news is that it is never too late to begin to fund this protection against retirement. Invest in yourself and one of the best ways to do this is through exercise.

Walking:

Walking is at a minimum of three times per week and preferably five to six. The goal is to walk 20 - 30 minutes per day. Initially, this could prove to be difficult. Therefore, we start with whatever you are comfortable with and then can increase in time and duration. This will help in building muscle strength, improving circulation and building neuronal connections.

If you are unable to walk, try a lower body ergometer, which you can pedal while you sit or perhaps a mini stair stepper that can be placed under your chair.

Stretching:

Stretching can be of benefit to improve circulation and muscle endurance. Stretching throughout the day, the calves, the legs, the back, shoulder, arms and wrist can help. If performed daily, this will also improve joint mobility and assist in the reduction of pain. The major muscle groups we recommend stretching are the hip flexors, hamstrings, quadriceps, and calves.

A simple stretch for the hip flexors, which get tight from sitting all day, is when you are on your bed in the supine position (nose up) then have your leg closest to the edge drop down off the bed and hold it for a count of 30 – 60 seconds. If this is easy for you then bring the opposite knee towards your chest.

The hamstring is the big muscle in the back of your thigh. There are several ways to stretch this muscle and I would recommend going online to look at all the options to see what is suitable in your daily routine. It can be stretched just by placing the leg in front of you and slowly begin to lean forward, if this does not hurt your back. There should be a gentle pull in the back of your thigh.

The quadriceps can be stretched by trying to bring your heel to your buttock while in the prone position (nose down).

To stretch the calves, we recommend leaning against a wall and placing one leg back. With the leg that is back, place some weight on the heel and you should feel a gentle stretch in the calf.

Doing figure 8's with your ankle is a nice easy way to gain mobility and improve circulation in the calves and ankles.

Stretching should always be done gently and make sure you breathe while you stretch.

Yoga / Chair Yoga

Yoga can also be helpful in its practices to help improve flexibility, reduces stress; minimize anxiety and the body's ability to tolerate pain. It works on important components of proper breathing, stretching and strengthening which can help with neuropathic pain. I recommend a beginner's class to start.

Chair Yoga is an easier way to perform the exercise adding value and benefit to the individual that is more sedentary and has difficulty moving around.

Tai Chi

Tai Chi is another exercise that I recommend to many of my neuropathy patients. It is a slow guided exercise that is very powerful to the cerebellum, which is the part of the brain that controls posture, balance and coordination.

In our office, we utilize stationary bicycles, vibrational platforms, foam stability pads, rocker boards, bosu- ball, TRX, and tubing exercises. It is important to enhance the cardiovascular system either through the recumbent bicycle or walking.

The benefits of exercise are well known and documented:

1. Reduce blood sugar levels.
2. Improve insulin resistance.
3. Improve strength and balance.

4. Lower fat levels.
5. Lower stroke risk.
6. Protect against Osteoporosis.

The less documented positive effects are:

1. Decreasing blood cortisol which is the stress hormone that increases fat storage.

2. Decreasing the sympathetic tone (fight or flight response).

3. Balancing hormone and neurotransmitter levels.

4. Increases angiogenesis (growth of new blood vessels)

5. Increase BDNF (Brain Derived Neurotrophic Factor) and the ability to establish new neuronal connections.

High Intensity Exercise

The key to a successful exercise program is to start slow and increase your intensity as your fitness level improves. To achieve the most beneficial results, it will be necessary to incorporate high intensity exercise 2-3 times per week. High intensity can best be described as, if you were working out, it would be difficult to carry out a conversation at the same time. If you are unable to speak at all then that is a little too much so decrease the intensity.

The bicycle is a good high intensity workout for peripheral neuropathy patients, since walking or the use of the treadmill could be irritating and painful.

It is important to measure your heart rate during the workouts and do not exceed the guideline of 180 – (your age).

For instance, if you are 68, the heart rate should not exceed 112, (180 – 68 = 112).

It has been proven that only 6 minutes of high intensity exercise is extremely beneficial to you. So, there are no more excuses that we do not have time to exercise. We all can find 6 minutes!

Vibration Therapy:

As I mentioned, we also love the vibration platform as a form of exercise in our office. First, this platform utilizes 95% of your muscle fibers. Secondly, it stimulates the large diameter afferent pathway in the body, which is extremely important for proprioception and inhibiting pain. To summarize, the vibrational platform will improve strength, proprioception, balance, and circulation and inhibit pain.

Typical Routine:

1. Chair squat: Use a safe sturdy chair, aim rear to the back of the chair. Keep chest up and push knees out. Squat slowly without using your hand, lowering your rear end to the chair. Notify your Doctor if you are having knee pain.
2. Push up or Wall Push up.
3. Horizontal Row.
4. Hip Abduction; Hip extension.
5. Clams.
6. Walking - build up to 30 minutes. Build up 5 to 10 minute intervals.
7. Bicycle or interval training – when you can work up to 30 minutes.

8. Vibration on the Calves and feet for approximately 5 - 10 minutes.

Beginner Routine:
1. Walk slow for 5 minutes.
2. Walk fast for 30 seconds.
3. Walk slow for 90 seconds.
4. Repeat 1 - 2 times.
5. Goal is to do this routine 7 times.

Before beginning any cardiovascular program, make sure you obtain approval from your doctor or cardiologist if you have a heart condition.

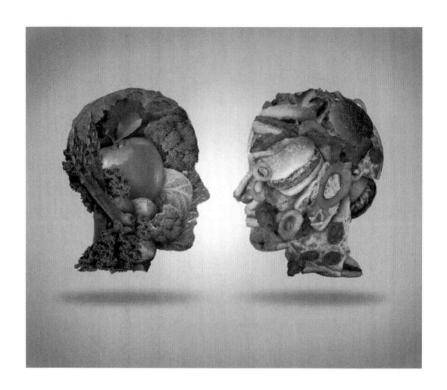

Chapter Twenty Five
DIET RECOMMENDATIONS

As we are all aware, there is a direct link between diet and health. We have learned that our dietary and lifestyle habits will affect our DNA and turn good genes on or bad genes off.

When it comes to Neuropathy, we talked in great length how high blood sugar and diabetes can be detrimental to the nerves and cause degeneration.

There are several other foods that we restrict because they can aggravate the nerves   These are:

146

1. Gluten, the protein in wheat has proven to be a factor in patients with neuropathy. Gluten is most commonly found in bread, pizza and pasta.

2. Casein, the protein found in dairy is highly inflammatory and can cause nerve pain. Most commonly, this is found in milk, cheese and butter.

3. Grains have a high glycemic index and hence raise the blood sugar too fast. These spikes create resistance over a period. Rice and cereals need to be avoided.

4. Sugar is hidden in many of our foods. It is imperative to look at the labels and identify the number of grams of sugar per serving.

5. Artificial Sweeteners such as Aspartame and MSG are excitotoxins and are not good for our nerves or nervous system. Sources of aspartame are diet sodas. Sources of MSG are canned goods and Asian foods. The food companies have also disguised MSG in food labels. If it contains glutamate, it is probably not so good for you.

6. Alcohol must be avoided. It is high in sugar content and creates stress on the liver which is our major organ of detoxification.

Foods That Benefit Neuropathy:

A diet high in green leafy vegetables is advisable.

Essential to nerve health are B Vitamins, Magnesium, Zinc and Vitamin D.

1. Vitamin B1 sources: navy bean, black beans, lentils and green peas

2. Vitamin B2 sources: spinach, asparagus, almonds, beet greens and soybeans

3. Vitamin B6 sources: tuna, beef, spinach, salmon and chicken

4. Vitamin B12 sources: salmon, tuna and yogurt

5. Vitamin D sources- salmon, yogurt and mushrooms

6. Magnesium sources: spinach, pumpkin seeds, quinoa and cashews

7. Zinc sources: shrimp, pumpkin seeds, sesame seeds and garbanzo beans

KETOGENIC BASICS

The primary objective of a ketogenic diet is to shift our body from a sugar burner as our primary source of energy into a fat burner.

This is accomplished by eating a low carbohydrate, moderate protein and high fat diet. Generally, we look for 65 - 80% of our calories from fat, 15 - 35% from protein and 5 - 15% from carbohydrates.

Clinically, this has proven to be very therapeutic for blood sugar regulation, memory and cognitive improvement, weight loss and slowing the aging process.

To put it simply, our brain and nerves love fat. In fact, studies have shown how it benefits Cardiovascular Disease, Metabolic Syndrome and Fatty Liver Disease.

To jump - start the body into a nutritional ketosis state, try and limit your carbohydrate intake to 20 - 25 grams. It is important to ensure that fat is your predominant source of calories and do not eat too much protein as this will convert to a sugar burning state.

I recommend eating good fat as well as maintaining good electrolyte balance. Here are some suggestions:

2 tablespoons of coconut oil or MCT oil per day.

2 tablespoons of organic grass-fed butter or ghee per day.

2 tablespoons of sea salt to be added to water throughout the day (good for electrolytes).

Food Ideas:

1. Fish and shellfish are Keto friendly foods
2. Low carbonation vegetables: these are the non-starchy vegetables
   a. Because of fiber content in vegetables, most carbonation have a very low net carbonation count. they generally range 0 - 8 grams per cup. So, fill your plate with veggies
3. Cheese: generally, only 1 gram of carbonation
4. Avocados: 2 net carbonation
5. Meat and chicken
6. Eggs
7. Coconut oil
8. Plain greek yogurt and cottage cheese
9. Olive oil
10. Nuts and seeds
11. Berries
12. Butter and cream
13. Shirataki noodles
14. Olives
15. Coffee and tea (unsweetened)
16. Dark chocolate and cocoa powder

There are apps on the market that help you keep track of fats, carbohydrates and proteins like myfitnesspal.com.

Paleo Diet:

The Paleo, or caveman diet as it has been called, is a good anti-inflammatory diet. It consists of any chicken, meat or fish, fruits and vegetables. Whole foods are recommended with no processed foods. Gluten, dairy, soy and sugar are to be avoided on the Paleo diet.

There is no diet that is perfect for each person. Some people love the ketogenic and have had fabulous results. There are others that prefer the Paleo or Mediterranean diet. We have had success with patients trending to a Vegan or Vegetarian type diet.

The most important part is discover what you are comfortable with and proceed. There are numerous recipes available online that provides great resources and support for Paleo and Ketogenic lifestyles.

A few are:

Thepaleomom.com

PaleOmg.com

Plantfriendlydiet.com

"Ketogenic Diet for Beginners" Facebook Page is an excellent reference.

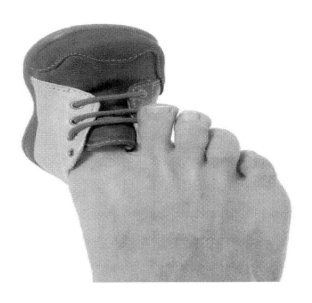

Chapter Twenty Six
FOOT WEAR/CARE

Foot Wear

It is often asked what type of shoe is the best for Neuropathy? This is a difficult question, but I have had more people endorse Sketchers, Birkenstocks and Uggs. Sketchers has a brand called Go Walk and Bobs, which are comfortable.

Some people state the inserts feel better and others feel it does not. Personally, I would not spend a lot of money on orthotics. I would purchase them on Amazon or CVS and get the inexpensive Dr. Scholl pads and try them. Sometimes, the hard orthotics is just too much on the feet.

Take Good Care of Your Feet

It is recommended that you check your feet daily. Look for cuts, blisters or swelling.

- Bathe feet daily in luke warm water.
- Moisturize feet but not between the toes as this could cause a fungal infection.
- Cut nails carefully.
- Keep feet warm and dry.

A few things I recommend for relief:

- Magnesium lotion by Life-Flo.
- Epsom salt baths.
- Roll with a massage stick on the calves and bottom of feet.
- Essential Oils: Essential Oils have proven to be effective in decreasing pain in the feet from peripheral neuropathy. In a study, 56 out of 60 individuals exhibited relief within 30 minutes. The blend was geranium, lavender, bergamot, tea tree and eucalyptus.
- EFAC cream or pills. I like to take the pills and cut them in half and rub the contents on the area of injury.
- Lidocaine creams have also proven to be beneficial to some patients.

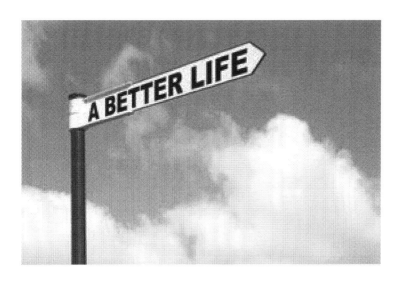

Chapter Twenty Seven
NEUROPATHY RECOVERY PROGRAM

Lifestyle Modifications:

The Essentials

Drink More Water: Our health is completely dependent upon water. We should drink approximately one half ounce of water for every pound of body weight per day. For example, if you weigh 150 pounds you should drink 75 ounces of water.

Pure spring water is the best. Coffee, tea, beer and soda dehydrate your body.

Just Breathe: Spend time focusing on your breathing taking deep breaths in and slowly exhaling. This will help deliver oxygen to your body to help it relax. Belly breathing is a proven technique to help calm your sympathetic tone (fight or flight) and increase Vagal Tone (rest and digest).

Belly Breathing Exercise

- Sit up straight and place your hands on your stomach.
- Breathe in, and concentrate on filing your stomach, not the chest. You should feel your hands on the belly rise and fall.
- Exhale slowly.
- Repeat this 8 - 10 slow deep breaths per minutes.

The exchange of oxygen and carbon dioxide is essential for mitochondrial health, cell energy and brain health.

Sleep: Our brain and immune system are dependent on a good night's sleep to stay healthy. Adults need approximately 7 - 8 hours per night. Here are some tips if you are having difficulty sleeping:

Begin to turn off all electronics one hour before bed, which includes TV, phone and computer. Darken the room to prevent any light from entering. This will stimulate melatonin production. Keep the cell phone and router out of the bedroom. Take an Epsom salt bath prior to bed to assist in the body's detoxification process.

If you fall asleep and wake up an hour or two later, address the gallbladder and stomach for proper digestion. **Sometimes,** eating a small amount of protein before bed will help you sleep through the night.

Smile and Laughter: A study published found that smiling reduced the heart rate and improved stressful recovery faster. Laughter will help to lower cortisol, our stress hormone, and boost endorphins, the "brain feel good" chemical. Laughter will also produce an opioid response in the brain.

Be Grateful and Give Thanks: I recommend keeping a journal and write down every day what you are thankful for. This simple act of gratitude and giving thanks helps focus your attention on something more positive and helps our difficulties appear to be less pronounced.

Meditate: Try meditating every day in a quiet room with no distractions. Let your thoughts and mind wander and focus on your breathing. Meditate in a position you feel most comfortable and focus on any one thing. Initially, it is difficult to be still but eventually you will adapt to this alpha state allowing your mind to relax.

Prayer: Praying for peace, serenity, gratitude with or without religious convictions will have a positive impact on your outlook, stress and pain.

Nature: Enjoy the simple things, spend time outside listening and watching the birds, gardening, taking photographs.

Eat More Whole Foods: Focus on eating real whole foods that are not processed and preferably organic. They are loaded with antioxidants, vitamins and minerals. Increase your intake of vegetables and fruits, nuts and seeds, and beans, which will increase your fiber intake and help regulate your blood sugar and lower cholesterol.

When you focus on eating whole foods, the paradigm shift changes from a diet mentality to a healthy lifestyle. This approach is sustainable especially when results begin to happen. This is when the magic begins and the change continues, and the overall health improves.

Movement: As we discussed in our section on exercise, movement is important for brain health, circulation and communication with neurons. It helps to stimulate the large diameter afferents providing constant communication to the brain and peripheral nervous system.

We are all aware of how detrimental the sedentary lifestyle is. However, sometimes it is very hard to make change. My recommendation would be to start slow and set goals every day of what you are going to accomplish with regards to not only exercise but also all the lifestyle and diet modifications we have discussed.

MINDFULNESS:

Mindfulness is a term used to describe living in the present or living in the "Now." The practice of mindfulness along with meditation can be very beneficial for many reasons.

- Manage Stress
- Manage Chronic Pain
- Balance "fight or flight"
- Reduce Anxiety

It is a state where we are completely 100% conscious and present in the moment in a non-judgmental manner. The effort is to quiet the mind, the internal dialogue that exists and to experience the pure quiet of being in that present moment.

Many studies have been done on the impact of the brain and the power of positive thinking and imagery. This state of mindfulness will stimulate the frontal lobes of the brain, and will stimulate the neurotransmitters dopamine and serotonin. These neurotransmitters affect our mood as well as behavior. Mindfulness will also stimulate GABA, the body's only inhibitor neurotransmitter and calms down norepinephrine.

Norepinephrine is responsible for regulating and monitoring the bodies stress response, Cortisol.

The frontal lobe has a tremendous impact on the body and it communicates directly to other parts of the brain including the basal ganglia and the thalamus. The basal ganglia can impact emotions and movement disorders such as tics and restless legs. The thalamus is important because this is the part of the brain that gaits pain and sensation.

Mindfulness mediation should be practiced on a daily basis for the chronic pain with neuropathy patient. Its benefits are substantial impacting your stress hormones, feel good hormones, the ability to gait the pain center as well as improving sleep.

When this is done in conjunction with the other ingredients we have discussed for improvement in your neuropathy symptoms, the results are much better. There must be a comprehensive plan, which incorporates the diet and lifestyle changes.

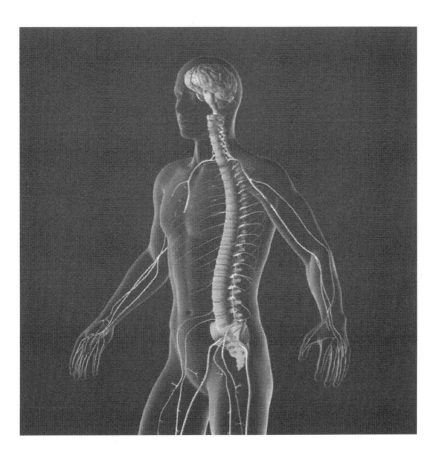

Chapter Twenty Eight
Can Nerves Regenerate?

The simple answer is "yes they have the ability to regenerate axons as long as the nerve itself has not died, which may lead to functional recovery over time. Correcting an underlying condition often can result in the neuropathy resolving on its own as the nerves recover or regenerate". This quote was taken from the National Institute of Neurological Disorders and Stroke.

To have success with the symptoms of neuropathy than the underlying cause has to be addressed, a complete examination must be performed and a proper treatment plan must be implemented.

Causes:

- Physical Injury: This can be caused by repetitive stress or trauma
- Metabolic or Endocrine: Diabetes, Hormone Imbalances, and Thyroid
- Autoimmunity: Rheumatoid Arthritis, Sjogren's, and Lupus
- Kidney or Liver Disease:
- Cancer and Chemo Induced Neuropathy
- Small Vessel Disease: Affecting oxygen to peripheral nerves
- Medication Toxicity
- Chemical Toxicity
- Vitamin Deficiencies
- Hereditary or Genetic Mutations: Charcot Marie Tooth
- Neuromas

Examination:

- Physical Examination
- Blood Work: CBC, Comprehensive Metabolic Panel, Nutrients
- Labs: Cyrex, Genova, Great Plains, Doctors Data, Genetics
- Testing: MRI, NCV, EMG
- Biopsy: Skin, Nerve

Plan:

- Dietary: Paleo, Ketogenic, Fodmaps
- Lifestyle: Exercise, Meditation, Prayer, Foot Wear/Care
- Supplements: Gut, Detoxification, Mitochondrial, Inflammation, Elimination
- Nerve Support: Specific nutrients researched to benefit nerve repair.
- Activation: Specific therapies and exercises designed to increase the BDNF which allows neurons to communicate with one another.

PERIPHERAL NEUROPATHY

NERVE DAMAGE

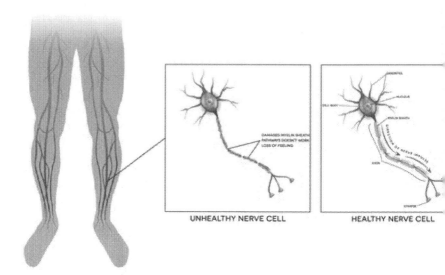

UNHEALTHY NERVE CELL   HEALTHY NERVE CELL

For a nerve to repair, it must be provided proper nutritional support. This nutritional support should not be taken without employing the other strategies we have outlined. It should incorporate the diet and lifestyle modifications. Otherwise, it is similar to throwing a dart and hoping for a bulls eye. For a minute, reflect on all the various supplements and creams you have purchased trying to find that relief.

It is time to go all in and begin to make the changes that are necessary for improvement.

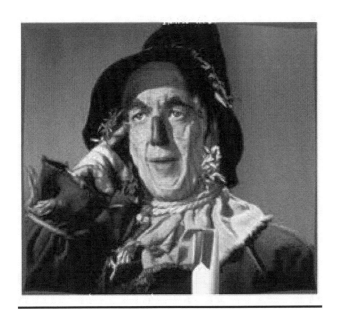

Chapter Twenty Nine
It's All In Your Head

"It's all in your head." I know at times we feel this way as we discuss the symptoms with the doctor and they give you a blank look like how can your vertigo, constipation, lack of motivation and foot tingling have any common ground. Even family members and friends have difficulty accepting how this all could be so real. How could there be something wrong with you when there is no visual evidence of an injury or pain.

In my opinion, the brain is the most overlooked aspect of neuropathy. In part, it is because we are just beginning to learn more about the brain, and its role in neuropathy. The concept of neuroplasticity has only been around since the early 1980's.

During this discussion, I am going to oversimplify the brain and how it interacts with neuropathy to open your eyes to another dimension that, perhaps, has been overlooked that could be affecting your symptoms.

First, we know the left side of the brain controls the right side of the body, and the right side of the brain controls the left side.

The part of the brain that is responsible for sensation is called the Parietal Lobe. Within the parietal lobe, there is a sensory strip, which controls sensation in different parts of the body.

They have completely mapped out the parts of the body within the parietal lobe, and this is called the homunculus.

Occasionally, the neuropathy can be an issue with the parietal lobe and its inability to interpret sensation properly.

If the neuropathy is on one side of the body, the parietal lobe certainly needs to be addressed.

Is it possible that a blow to the head in the parietal lobe could affect you later in life?

Another part of the brain that I believe is extremely important with Neuropathy is the Cerebellum. This has often been called the second brain. The cerebellum's function is balance, posture and coordination. It is by far the most dependent part of the body for oxygen and glucose. As stated earlier, every neuron to function properly needs glucose, oxygen and activation. If we have glucose issues, anemia, COPD, or even sleep apnea, this can affect the cerebellum as well as other parts of the brain.

There has also been a lot of research on how gluten, dairy and alcohol can affect the cerebellum. That is why we recommend to avoid gluten, dairy and alcohol on the anti-inflammatory diet.

I am often asked "did my neuropathy cause the balance issue?"

This is a difficult question, since no two people are the same with their cause of neuropathy and their symptoms. I will say the cerebellum certainly needs to be addressed and improved if the neuropathy is going to improve.

The Frontal lobe is another important part of the brain that often gets ignored with neuropathy. It contains most of the dopamine sensitive neurons associated with short term memory, motivation, and executive function like planning, attention and reward.

For a long time, there has been agreement that Restless Legs Syndrome is the result of too much dopamine and how it interacts with another part of the brain called the basal ganglia. However, new research is pointing towards glutamate and its role in restless legs syndrome.

Glutamate is necessary to make our only inhibitory neurotransmitter, GABA. However, due to a genetic inability to break glutamate down properly with the GAD enzyme, glutamate can build up in the system creating hyper movement disorders.

The second reason, which is a bit more frightening, is that some of the food companies place or hide glutamates in our foods. Since we became fairly knowledgeable about the pitfalls of MSG (monosodium glutamate), they decided to change the names to hide the identity of MSG. This is another reason why I recommend whole foods and no processed foods.

If you are having issues with Restless Legs Syndrome, Google hidden names with MSG, and start to read the labels and avoid consuming those foods.

The Temporal Lobe of the brain is very important for a few reasons. First, this is where our hearing and sense of smell is located. Second, this is where the hippocampus is located and it converts short term memory to long term memory. The hippocampus is what gets affected in Alzheimer's and Dementia.

The lobes of the brain along with the cerebellum have a feedback loop to the brainstem and mid brain which keeps our fight or flight response in check. If there is dysfunction in any part of the brain or inflammation then this feedback system becomes affected and we begin to lose the brake pedal. Symptoms like heart rate, respiration, blood pressure and sleep can be affected.

What also will become affected is the Vagus Nerve, the rest and digest nerve. When our body becomes dominant in the sympathetic tone, the parasympathetic part of the nervous system begins to take the hit.

The Vagus nerve is responsible for motility, digestion, and sleep. It also helps control the HCL production in the gut that allows us to break down the food we eat properly. If this is not healthy, situations like Candida overgrowth, SIBO (small intestine bacterial overgrowth), or even bloating after a meal can occur.

I attribute much of the success we have had with improving Peripheral Neuropathy symptoms to the comprehensive approach we employ. This includes activation of the nerves, improving circulation, brain stimulation through various exercises, diet and nutritional supplementation and lifestyle modifications as we discussed.

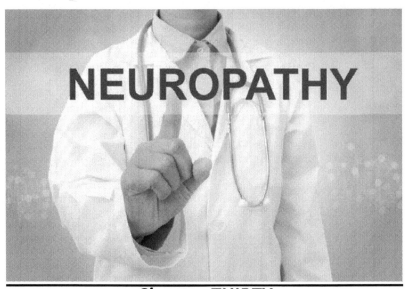

Chapter *THIRTY*
OUR FOCUS

There are no two patients that begin our program that are similar in the causes of neuropathy and inflammation. Our goal is to treat the whole person and restore their lives so that they can enjoy their daily activities, as they should.

A personalized treatment program is developed so that recovery and improvement can become a possibility.

We should not categorize all neuropathy patients into one block and assume that the individual with diabetic neuropathy should be treated the same as chemo induced neuropathy or an autoimmune condition such as sjogren's.

Our success has been determined by adherence to these principles. Discover the underlying cause of the problem and not just treat the symptoms.

Inflammation is the most common thread we have seen with all our chronic conditions. This affects the neurological system as well as the metabolic system. The most common causes are blood sugar abnormalities, anemia, autoimmunity and food sensitivities.

When these causes remain unchecked, the inflammatory process begins this cascade of events that leads to leaky gut and other peripheral symptoms.

With our remove, repair, replace and rejuvenate approach, we can minimize or eliminate the inflammatory process and therefore reducing the degree of nerve degeneration.

To stimulate the peripheral nerves to regenerate, we utilize many therapies dependent on the patient. We like electric muscle stimulation with a very specific waveform, which has been proven that this signal is unique to peripheral nerves.

We also utilize infrared therapy and cold laser for certain local peripheral entrapment or neuropathy issues.

As discussed, we recommend advanced nutritional supplementation along with exercise therapy done in the office and home to restore the nerve function and improve muscle balance and coordination.

If I was asked the question 10 years ago, "Can neuropathy be controlled or reversed?", my answer would have been, emphatically, NO. Neuropathy is a progressive disease and, if not controlled, it will continue to get worse. With the emergence of treatment modalities and the inclusion of a whole person approach, neuropathy can be controlled, and I have clinically seen numerous cases of improvement.

There is no cure for neuropathy but there is a lot of room for improvement given the right tools to improve the fuel, activation and delivery system.

The magic lotion, potion or pill generally will not work. With neuropathy, all aspects outlined in this book need to be addressed.

Each patient must be addressed structurally, metabolically and neurologically. With this formula, we have witnessed success with the intensity, frequency and duration from the symptoms of neuropathy.

A patient's success is dependent on them working with a doctor that understands the complexities of neuropathy, and how to control the metabolic and neurological issues.

The nerves will begin to regenerate once the driving source of inflammation is eliminated, nutritional deficiencies are addressed, the correct modality of treatment is prescribed, and the home exercises are performed.

In my 30 years of practice, I have seen a lot of changes, but peripheral neuropathy was the one condition that was always the most difficult to manage and treat. Now, when asked if it can be controlled or improved my answer would be, YES.

We have been fortunate to help change the lives of several of our patients with our Peripheral Neuropathy Recovery Program. Thank you, again, to the patients, you know who you are, that kept me on target and to the people that paved the way to make learning enjoyable and recovery a possibility.

"We got this."

GLYCEMIC INDEX OF FOODS

FOOD	GLYCEMIC INDEX	RATING
Bakery Products/Breads		
Soya and Linseed	36	Low
Wholegrain Pumpernickel	46	Low
Heavy mixed grain	45	Low
Whole wheat	49	Low
Sourdough Rye	48	Low
Sourdough wheat	54	Low
100% whole grain	51	Low
Corn tortilla	52	Low
Wheat tortilla	30	Low
Croissant	67	Med
Hamburger bun	61	Med
Pita, white	68	Med
Waffles, Aunt Jemima	76	High
Baguette, white, plain	95	High
Kaiser role	73	High

White wheat flour bread	71	High
Wonder bread	73	High
Whole wheat bread, average	71	High
Bagel, white, average	72	High
Beverages		
Tomato juice, canned	38	Low
Orange juice, unsweetened	50	Low
Apple juice, unsweetened	44	Low
Coca Cola, average	63	Med
Cranberry juice, cocktail	68	Med
Gatorade	78	High
Breakfast Cereals & related products		
All-Bran, average	55	Low
Oatmeal	55	Low
Natural Muesli	40	Low
Mini Wheats	58	Med
Nurtrigrain	66	Med
Cream of Wheat	66	Med
Raisin Bran	61	Med

Cheerios	74	High
Rice Krispies	82	High
FOOD	**GLYCEMIC INDEX**	**RATING**
Grains/Staples		
Quinoa	53	Low
Brown Rice, average	50	Low
Wheat pasta shapes	54	Low
Spaghetti	32	Low
White Long Grain Rice	50	Low
Sweet Potatoes	48	Low
Tortellini (cheese)	50	Low
Basmati Rice	58	Med
Couscous	65	Med
Sweet corn on the cob	60	Med
Baked potatoes	60	Med
Cornmeal	68	Med
Instant white rice	87	High
Fresh mashed potatoes	73	High
French Fries	75	High
Legumes (beans) and Nuts		
Baked beans	40	Low
Blackeye peas	33	Low

Black beans	30	Low
Peanuts	13	Low
Walnuts	15	Low
Nuts and Raisins	21	Low
Cashews	27	Low
Soy beans	15	Low
Kidney beans	29	Low
Vegetables		
Frozen green peas	39	Low
Frozen sweet corn	47	Low
Raw carrots	16	Low
Eggplant	15	Low
Broccoli	10	Low
Cauliflower	15	Low
Cabbage	10	Low
Mushrooms	10	Low
Tomatoes	15	Low
Chilies	10	Low
Lettuce	10	Low
Green beans	15	Low
Red peppers	10	Low
Onions	10	Low

Beetroot	64	Med
Pumpkin	75	High
Parsnips	97	High
FOOD	**GLYCEMIC INDEX**	**RATING**
Fruits		
Cherries	22	Low
Plums	24	Low
Grapefruit	25	Low
Peaches	28	Low
Apples	34	Low
Pears	41	Low
Dried Apricots	32	Low
Grapes	43	Low
Coconut milk	41	Low
Kiwi fruit	47	Low
Oranges	40	Low
Strawberries	40	Low
Prunes	29	Low
Mango	60	Med
Bananas	58	Med
Raisins	64	Med
Papaya	60	Med

Pineapple	66	Med
Watermelon	80	High
Dates	103	High
Dairy		
Whole milk	31	Low
Skimmed milk	32	Low
Chocolate milk	42	Low
Reduced fat yogurt, w/ fruit	33	Low
Soy milk	44	Low
Ice cream	62	Med
Cookies/Crackers & Snacks		
Snickers bar (high fat)	41	Low
Nut & Seed Muesli Bar	49	Low
Nutella	33	Low
Milk Chocolate	42	Low
Corn chips	42	Low
Oatmeal crackers	55	Low
Blueberry muffin	59	Med
Honey	58	Med
Rye crisps, average	64	Med
Shortbread	64	Med

Graham crackers	74	High
Rice cakes	82	High
Soda crackers	74	High
Pretzels	8 3	High

REFERENCES

Effects of methylcobalamin on diabetic neuropathy.
Yaqub BA, Siddique A, Sulimani R.Clin Neurol Neurosurg. 1992; 94(2):105-11.

Vitamin B12 may be more effective than nortriptyline in improving painful diabetic neuropathy.
Talaei A, Siavash M, Majidi H, Chehrei A.Int J Food Sci Nutr. 2009; 60 Suppl 5:71-6. Epub 2009 Feb 11.

Effectiveness of vitamin B12 on diabetic neuropathy: systematic review of clinical controlled trials.
Sun Y, Lai MS, Lu CJ.Acta Neurol Taiwan. 2005 Jun; 14(2):48-54.

Meta-analysis of methylcobalamin alone and in combination with lipoic acid in patients with diabetic peripheral neuropathy.

Xu Q, Pan J, Yu J, Liu X, Liu L, Zuo X, Wu P, Deng H, Zhang J, Ji A.Diabetes Res Clin Pract. 2013 Aug; 101(2):99-105. Epub 2013 May 9.

The peripheral neuropathy evaluation in an office-based neurology setting.
Vavra MW, Rubin DI.Semin Neurol. 2011 Feb; 31(1):102-14. Epub 2011 Feb 14.

Paraesthesia and peripheral neuropathy.
Beran R.Aust Fam Physician. 2015 Mar; 44(3):92-5.

Diabetic peripheral neuropathy and the management of diabetic peripheral neuropathic pain.
Morales-Vidal S, Morgan C, McCoyd M, Hornik A.Postgrad Med. 2012 Jul; 124(4):145-   53.

The evaluation of peripheral neuropathy. Part II: Identifying common clinical syndromes.
Kelly JJ.Rev Neurol Dis. 2004 Fall; 1(4):190-201.

Alpha-lipoic acid in the treatment of diabetic peripheral and cardiac autonomic neuropathy.
Ziegler D, Gries FA.Diabetes. 1997 Sep; 46 Suppl 2:S62-6.

The relationship between vitamin D status and cardiac autonomic neuropathy in patients with type 2 diabetes mellitus.
Jung CH, Jung SH, Kim KJ, Kim BY, Kim CH, Kang SK, Mok JO.Diab Vasc Dis Res. 2015 Sep; 12(5):342-51. Epub 2015 Jul 6.

Charcot Marie Tooth disease: principles of rehabilitation, physiotherapy and occupational therapy].
Sautreuil P, Delorme D, Baron A, Mane M, Missaoui B, Thoumie P.Med Sci (Paris). 2017 Nov; 33 Hors série n°1:49-54. Epub 2017 Nov 15.

Effect of Mindfulness-Based Stress Reduction vs Cognitive Behavioral Therapy or Usual Care on Back Pain and Functional Limitations in Adults With Chronic Low Back Pain: A Randomized Clinical Trial.
Cherkin DC, Sherman KJ, Balderson BH, Cook AJ, Anderson ML, Hawkes RJ, Hansen KE, Turner JA.JAMA. 2016 Mar 22-29; 315(12):1240-9.

Agelink MW, Malessa R, Weisser U, et al. Alcoholism, peripheral neuropathy (PNP) and cardiovRandomized Trial of the Effect of Mindfulness-Based Stress Reduction on Pain-Related Disability, Pain Intensity, Health-Related Quality of Life, and A1C in Patients With Painful Diabetic Peripheral Neuropathy. The Therapeutic Potential of Monocyte/Macrophage Manipulation in the Treatment of Chemotherapy-Induced Painful Neuropathy.

Progressive degeneration of motor nerve terminals in GAD mutant mouse with hereditary sensory axonopathy.*Miura H, Oda K, Endo C, Yamazaki K, Shibasaki H, Kikuchi T.Neuropathol Appl Neurobiol. 1993 Feb; 19(1):41-51.*

Old or new medicine? Vitamin B12 and peripheral nerve neuropathy].
Tanaka H.Brain Nerve. 2013 Sep; 65(9):1077-82

Methylcobalamin: a potential vitamin of pain killer.
Zhang M, Han W, Hu S, Xu H.Neural Plast. 2013; 2013:424651. Epub 2013 Dec 26.

Alpha-Lipoic acid: a metabolic antioxidant which regulates NF-kappa B signal transduction and protects against oxidative injury.
Packer L.Drug Metab Rev. 1998 May; 30(2):245-75.

Alpha-lipoic acid increases Na+K+ATPase activity and reduces lipofuscin accumulation in discrete brain regions of aged rats.
Arivazhagan P, Panneerselvam C.Ann N Y Acad Sci. 2004 Jun; 1019:350-4.

Dual effects of antioxidants in neurodegeneration: direct neuroprotection against oxidative stress and indirect protection via suppression of glia-mediated inflammation.
Wang JY, Wen LL, Huang YN, Chen YT, Ku MC.Curr Pharm Des. 2006; 12(27):3521-33

Vitamin B for treating peripheral neuropathy.
Ang CD, Alviar MJ, Dans AL, Bautista-Velez GG, Villaruz-Sulit MV, Tan JJ, Co HU, Bautista MR, Roxas AA.Cochrane Database Syst Rev. 2008 Jul 16; (3):CD004573. Epub 2008 Jul 16.

Benfotiamine in the treatment of diabetic polyneuropathy--a three-week randomized, controlled pilot study (BEDIP study).
Haupt E, Ledermann H, Köpcke W.Int J Clin Pharmacol Ther. 2005 Feb; 43(2):71-7.

Behse F, Buchthal F. Alcohol Neuropathy: Clinical, Electrophysiological and Biopsy Findings. *Ann Neurol*. 1977;2:95-10.

Brust JCM, Britton C, Chiriboga CA, et al. In: Mancall EL, ed. Neurological Complications of Substance Abuse. *Vol3*. 1997:89.

Hillbom M, Wennberg A. Prognosis of alcoholic peripheral neuropathy. *J Neurol Neurosurg Psychiatry*. Jul 1984;47(7):699-703

Johnson RH, Robinson BJ. Mortality in alcoholics with autonomic neuropathy. *J Neurol NeurosurgPsychiatry*. Apr 1988;51(4):476-80.

Kharbanda PS, Prabhakar S, Chawla YK. Peripheral neuropathy in liver cirrhosis. *J Gastroenterol Hepatol*. Aug 2003;18(8):922-926.

Monforte R, Estruch R, Valls-Sole J, et al. Autonomic and peripheral neuropathies in patients with chronic alcoholism. A dose-related toxic effect of alcohol. *Arch Neurol*. Jan 1995;52(1):45-51.]

Beggs, S., Liu, X.J., Kwan, C., Salter, M.W., 2010. Peripheral nerve
injury and TRPV1-expressing primary afferent C-fibers cause opening of the blood-brain barrier. Mol. Pain 6, 74.
Benn, S.C., Perrelet, D., Kato, A.C., Scholz, J., Decosterd, I., Mannion,
R.J., Bakowska, J.C., Woolf, C.J., 2002. Hsp27 upregulation and

Martyn C, Hughes R. Epidemiology of peripheral neuropathy. J Neurol & Neurosur

Sabin T, Swift T, Jacobson R. Leprosy. In: Dyck PJ, Thomas PK, editors. Peripheral
neuropathy. Philadelphia: WB Saunders; 1993. p. 1354–79.

Asbury A, Gilliatt R. The clinical approach to neuropathy. In: Asbury A, Gilliat R,
editors. Peripheral nerve disorders: a practical approach. London: Butterworths; 1984. p.
1–20.

McLeod J, Tuck R, Pollard J, Cameron J, Walsh J. Chronic polyneuropathy of undetermined
cause. J Neurol Neurosurg Psychiatry 1984;47:530–5.

Dyck PJ, Dyck PJ, Grant IA, Fealey RD. Ten steps in characterizing and diagnosing
patients with peripheral neuropathy. Neurology 1996;47:10–7.

Morgenlander JC. Recognizing peripheral neuropathy. How to read the clues and
underlying cause. Postgrad Med 1997;102:71–80.

Donofrio PD, Albers JW. AAEM minimonograph #34: Polyneuropathyclassification by
nerve conduction studies and electromyography. Muscle Nerve 1990;13:889–902.

Lubec D, Mullbacher W, Finsterer J, Mamoli B. Diagnostic work-up in peripheral neuropathy:
an analysis of 171 cases. Postgrad Med J 1999;75:723–7.

Barohn RJ. Approach to peripheral neuropathy and neuronopathy. Semin Neurol 1998;
18:7–18.

Bosch EP, Mitsumoto H. Disorders of peripheral nerve. In: Bradley WG, Daroff RB,
Fenichel GM, Marsden CD, editors. Neurology in clinical practice. Boston: Butterworth-
Heinemann; 1996. p. 1881–1952.

Poncelet AN. An algorithm for the evaluation of peripheral neuropathy. American Family Physician 1998;15:755–64.

Sabin T. Classification of peripheral neuropathy: the long and the short of it. Muscle Nerve 1986;9:711–719.

Chaudhry V. Multifocal motor neuropathy. Semin Neurol 1998;18:73–81.

] Taylor B, Wright R, Harper C, Dyck P. Natural history of 46 patients with multifocal
motor neuropathy with conduction block. Muscle Nerve 2000;23:900–8.

] Albers JW. Toxic Neuropathies. In Bromberg M. (Director). Peripheral Neuropathy.
Philadelphia, PA: American Academy of Neurology Course 2FC.004, May 6, 2001.

Research criteria for diagnosis of chronic inflammatory demyelinating polyneuropathy
(CIDP). Report from an Ad Hoc Subcommittee of the American Academy of Neurology
AIDS Task Force. Neurology 1991;41:617–8.

Meulstee J, van der Mech FG. Electrodiagnostic criteria for polyneuropathy and demyelination:
application in 135 patients with Guillain-Barre syndrome. Dutch Guillain-Barre
Study Group. J Neurol Neurosurg Psychiatry. 1995;59:482–6.

Portenoy RK. Painful polyneuropathy. Neurol Clin 1989;7:265–8.

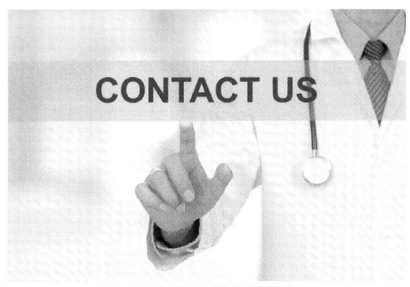

COACHING PROGRAM

If you are interested in our coaching program to help guide you through this complex maze, go to our website drmichaelveselak.com. We are accustomed to working with distance patients.

We offer an online step by step process for the neuropathy recovery program. This includes tutorials on dietary recommendations with meal plans and specific exercises designed to improve nerve function. Proper supplementation and email support.

There is no program like this that will guide you through the entire process.

Additional Resources

The Neuropathy Association
60 E. 42nd Street, Suite 942
New York, Ny 10165
Http://www.neuropathy.org

American Chronic Pain Association
P.O. Box 850
Rocklin, CA 95677
Http://www.theacpa.org

Join Us

Facebook: Chronic Pain: Understanding, Managing and Improving Neuropathy and Fibromyalgia.

We will be answering questions about the book and having facebook live videos about some of the topics discussed. This will be a closed group. Share, discuss and, show support with other Neuropathy Warriors.

Made in the USA
Middletown, DE
04 January 2020